Praise for *Barefoot Running*

Dear Readers, enjoy the insights this book has to offer to help you to remember to run in an easy, light, and smooth way, with or without footwear of your choice. It is about form, joy, and the love of running. Run free!

—Micah True, Caballo Blanco de la Sierra Madre

Barefoot Running is the best book on the market on how to begin and excel at barefoot running. I highly recommend it.

—Dr. Michael Nirenberg, podiatric physician and surgeon,
and author of America's Podiatrist Blog

Barefoot Running arrives on the crest of a major paradigm shift in the world of running as, once again, we come to realize that nature is indeed best. Michael Sandler's exhaustive treatment of the topic celebrates the amazing evolutionary success that is the human foot and serves as a comprehensive user's guide for its rehabilitation and proper maintenance.

—Dr. Joseph Froncioni, MDCM, FRCS(C)

As Michael Sandler argues compellingly, there are lots of good neurological reasons to re-attach yourself to the holy ground that you walk on!

If predictability and reliability in the contact of your feet to the ground was a good thing, human evolution would have provided us with hooves! Reconnecting with the irregular earth for at least a short period of time every day is definitely good for both your brain AND body!

Taking off those shoes, walking on a natural landscape where each step can provide a surprise, and feeling the earth between your toes for at least a short time every day is a very good idea, for brain and body alike!

—Michael M. Merzenich, Ph.D., Director of Scientific Learning Corporation,
Francis A. Sooy Chair of Otolaryngology in the Keck Center for Integrative
Neurosciences at the University of California, San Francisco Medical Center

The history of running comes full circle with the publication of *Barefoot Running*. Michael Sandler and Jessica Lee join the ranks of Dean Karnazes and Christopher McDougall as prophets of running in the 21st century, showing us how to be smarter, lighter and better runners, just as our first ancestors were so many millenia ago. Any runner wanting to run with better form will like this book.

—Michael Sandrock, author of *Running with the Legends*,
and founder of One World Running

I'm often asked where to start. Now I can say, start here.

—Marc Richard Silberman, MD
Director, New Jersey Sports Medicine and Performance Center

Michael and Jessica have provided a guide to help you avoid and minimize the problems associated with awakening your feet and your body, by embracing your bare feet. The question is no longer, should we be barefoot? It is, how often, and how much? *Barefoot Running* is the best current synopsis of the evidence of the benefits of aware feet, and the most logical guide to attaining them.

—Ray McClanahan, DPM, BS Ed, creator of Correct Toes,
and founder of Northwest Foot & Ankle Clinic

For all the hi-tech innovations of the running shoe industry in the past decades, the truth is finally catching on. Nature has provided us with a feat of engineering so magnificent that it could never be replicated by science—a pair of feet. In their natural state they are perfectly suited to running, and yet for many runners, particularly in the Western world, they have been devalued, underutilized, misused, and abused. The definitive user's manual—*Barefoot Running*—has finally been written. Sell your shoes, buy the book, and let your feet take you on breathtaking adventures previously undreamed of.

—Lorraine Mueller, four-time Olympian, Marathon Bronze Medalist,
and author of *On the Wings of Mercury*

Michael Sandler's experience and research gives any runner vital information on how to run healthier for decades, whether you choose to wear shoes or not. His principles and teaching on how the foot and body all work in proper anatomic function and how to correct dysfunctions is vitally important for running health and performance. I have been applying these principles for 10 years now, have not had injury, and still continue to run marathons in under 2:35 at age 43. Like Michael, I was told not to run 10 years ago after operations on my feet. You too can be your own coach armed with the right knowledge.

—Mark Cucuzzella, MD, Associate Professor of Family Medicine,
West Virginia University School of Medicine
Race Director, Freedom's Run and owner of Two Rivers Treads

The research is out and the evidence is clear that barefoot running puts less stress and strain on your joints than running in footwear. Michael Sandler's book, *Barefoot Running*, will teach you step-by-step how to transition from shod running back to natural running safely and effectively.

—Dr. James Stoxen, DC, President of Team Doctors,
and member of the National Fitness Hall of Fame

BAREFOOT RUNNING

BAREFOOT RUNNING

How to Run Light and Free by Getting in Touch with the Earth

MICHAEL SANDLER
with Jessica Lee
Co-founders, RunBare Company

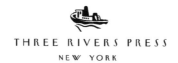

THREE RIVERS PRESS
NEW YORK

Originally published by
RunBare Publishing, in Boulder, CO, in 2010.

Library of Congress Cataloging-in-Publication Data is available upon request.

ISBN 978-0-307-98593-4
eISBN 978-0-307-98594-1

Printed in the United States of America on 20% recycled paper

Editor: Sandra Wendel, Write On, Inc.
Cover photograph: Kennan Harvey, Kennan Harvey Photography
Cover design by Gregory Fields and James Massey
Book design by Gregory Fields, www.fieldsgraphics.com
Studio photography: Josephine Pham, J.Pham Photography
Outdoor photography: Jessica Lee and Michael Sandler
Running stick man: Jessica Lee and Michael Sandler

1 3 5 7 9 10 8 6 4 2

First Three Rivers Press Edition

Dedication

I opened up my eyes and there you were.

You opened up my eyes and here we are.

When I started barefoot running a few years ago, it was only to heal. I was told I could no longer run, and couldn't accept that. Once I went barefoot, everything changed. I went from constantly injured and running meek, to dancing on the trails and flying on the roads.

I've coached athletes for the better part of 20 years. Yet until I met Jessica Lee, the idea of teaching barefoot running never occurred to me. One day the *Denver Post* came out to photograph me chasing down cyclists, uphill barefoot and it dawned on Jessica that I had an important story to share. Then she told us we should start a club. That club quickly grew to hundreds of members, dozens at a time showing up for our clinics. Then she said we should start a business, RunBare Company, and that began to take off. And then she said we should write this book.

None of this, from the club, to RunBare Company, to this book, our massive tour, clinics, products, reviews, you-name-it, would have existed without her. She opened up my eyes, and I'm forever thankful, and so I dedicate this book to her.

I also dedicate this book to Pumpkin and Sawa, our two four-leggers or little girls—puppies at any age who've been the ultimate barefooters and have guided me and brightened our lives with their smiles, energy, and pure love of running.

—Michael Sandler

I opened Michael's eyes, but God opened mine.

It's difficult for me to take credit for coming up with the ideas that Michael mentions, starting a club, a business and writing a book. These ideas sort of bubbled up out of nowhere. They came to me at odd times, once while cooking eggs for breakfast, through conversations with friends, but often in meditations. Yet with the upsurge in popularity for barefoot running, the timing was perfect. The plan was perfect, a perfection neither Michael nor I are capable of. All I knew was, together, Michael and I could help a lot of people and the doors kept opening. Our job in essence was quite simple. All we had to do was to keep faith and continue stepping through the doors into the unknown.

Admittedly, doubts and fears arose, challenges that required what we so often called "squeezing through tight and narrow doorways." And here's where great teamwork came in. Michael was a constant reminder that anything is possible, as demonstrated by his belief that he would walk and even run again following his near-death accident. Though I'm apt to call him a "cheese ball," Michael reminds me to witness the beauty of the world around me and the miracles that occur each and every day.

Our vision is simple. To help as many people as we can. What that looks like, we'll only see when we arrive in the moment. We plan, we want to control, but in the end we have to let go. Ultimately, it's not our plan. It's a delicate balance and one of the greatest lessons of our lifetimes.

Thank you God for bringing Michael into my life and for guiding us on this miraculous journey.

—Jessica Lee

Contents

Special Greeting from Barefoot Ted

I've often called Christopher McDougall's book *Born to Run* my quirky Ph.D. thesis I didn't have to write. He was able to take everything I had learned about the fundamental human capacity of running, joyfully and minimally, and turn it into an epic book that has changed the thinking of a generation.

Michael Sandler's book continues that theme.

Thousands upon thousands of folks have contacted me asking how they too can begin their barefoot journey. My solution has been to conduct introductory clinics to barefoot running and to share my stories on my blog Barefoot Ted's Adventures. Many encourage me to write a how-to book about barefoot running.

Now I don't have to write that book either. Here it is.

Michael Sandler has applied his passion and insights into barefoot running in a way no one else has so far. You are holding in your hands a book as exhaustive and accurate of a description of barefoot running as you could ever hope for.

I am proud of this book's message and its attention to detail and quality of writing. I dare to say that this book will become a best-seller and inform millions about the benefits of barefoot running—and not just the physical benefits. Michael touches on the deeper, spiritual aspects of running and our deep connection with the earth, our ancestors, and all the other co-inhabitants on this planet. You will be inspired.

Once again the Universe has been generous to me and you and found someone who could thoughtfully and exhaustively write about a topic that will ultimately change the lives of all who read it and practice what it teaches.

You are a very lucky person. You were born with amazing capacities that are waiting reawakening. Taking off your shoes is a first big step.

—Barefoot Ted

Barefoot Ted's Adventures
www.BarefootTed.com

Foreword

by Danny Dreyer
Coauthor of *ChiRunning*

Looking back on my childhood there were two days every year that will always stand out in my memory—one was my favorite and the other my least favorite.

My favorite day was the last day of school. I'd sit in class and count down the hours and minutes until that last bell rang because I knew it meant the freedom of summer vacation. I wouldn't have to sit at a desk all day, and I could play to my heart's content—and *I didn't have to wear shoes for three months*—until my least favorite day. Back to school in the fall. The only time I was required to wear shoes was to go to church, when I had to wear those torturous ill-begotten things called "dress shoes."

I remember ritually throwing away my "school" shoes on the last day of school and relishing the delightful sense of feeling the ground again. My feet were tender at first, but I knew that within days I'd be running around, playing with my friends.

Those first few barefoot days were rough, but there was no way around it. When I wanted to go over to my best friend's house to play, I'd walk along seeking out every patch of grass I could find. Gradually my feet would become more accustomed to the hardness of the streets and sidewalks, and eventually, I could handle even gravel roads. But all that was worth it because my whole body felt such joy without shoes.

Late in those hot August days, with September fast approaching, I began to dread putting shoes on again. My mother would always buy me a new pair for the school year, and when I'd first put them on, they felt so clunky and stiff, and just plain weird. I felt blocked from feeling the dirt between my toes. I couldn't run and jump as easily, and I certainly couldn't move as fast. The days of footloose freedom were over, and I began my countdown to summer once again.

This repeating cycle of shod and unshod continued until middle school when I began to do summer jobs, most of which required wearing shoes. Inevitably, through the subsequent years I became more used to always wearing shoes, and I just accepted it as part of being an adult.

My story might sound familiar to you. If it does and you miss that sense of connection with the earth under your feet, you'll appreciate this book. Michael Sandler and Jessica Lee have done a fabulous job of "reintroducing" us to barefooting, and we all have a lot to regain from this current "back to the future movement."

That being said, I'm beginning to see even greater importance that going barefoot can have on us as a society. Consider this:

The 1950s started the Age of Convenience with a multitude of inventions designed to give Americans more free time—the pop-up toaster, the modern refrigerator, TV, washers and dryers, jet passenger planes, Veg-a-matics and more.

Then came the '60s and '70s and the dawning of the Age of Technology with computers, mobile telephones, wireless remote controls, pagers, and the first video games. Through the '80s and '90s we saw the boom of cell phones and personal computers and the Information Age in which we now have instant search-engine access to answers for almost any question … except maybe, "How can I stay grounded in the midst of all of this?"

We've spent the better part of the last 60 years evolving a lifestyle that has left us increasingly desensitized to the earth we live on. No doubt about it, we've become a society of talking heads that drift from one text message, email, or cell phone call to the next. It seems more fashionable to text or tweet than to talk in person. We engage in behavior patterns that cut us off from our bodies, and the vast majority of us are in desperate need of a convenient and easy way to reconnect with our bodies.

I'd have to say that the quickest and most effective way to balance out being stuck in your head is to direct your awareness to the place in your body that is the farthest from your head—to the soles of your feet.

Walking or running barefoot on a daily basis is the perfect antidote for a culture desperately needing to find balance and grounding. Barefoot running and walking is free. It's easy. It doesn't take much time out of your day. And this is my favorite part: we have all loved going barefoot at some point in our lives, so there are no excuses.

There's a revolution afoot … so pass the word.

Danny Dreyer, Founder of ChiRunning
and Coauthor with his wife, Katherine, of
ChiRunning: A Revolutionary Approach to Effortless, Injury-free Running and
ChiWalking: Fitness Walking for Lifelong Health and Energy
www.ChiRunning.com

BAREFOOT RUNNING

Introduction

I fell into barefoot running entirely by accident—literally.

On April second of 2006 I was injured in a near-death accident.

I'd been skating on a local bike path as I trained for a world-record attempt, a 4,000-mile, solo coast-to-coast skate to help children with learning disabilities and attention deficit disorder. I'd done a similar journey in 2004, a 5,000 mile, 40-day, solo, unsupported bike ride across the U.S., which got me invited to speak in Washington, D.C., before the House and Senate.

On this day I had taken off my skates to meditate in the river, clear my mind, and pray for safety and guidance. Then I laced up my skates and pushed off. I'd been listening to Dr. Wayne Dyer's audiobook *Inspiration* on my MP3 player. He'd just shared a beautiful story about a butterfly that landed in his hands, before saying "everything happens for a reason."

As I began skating again, I told myself to go slow, aware that on Sundays there would be tourists on the path. What happened next, I didn't expect. A tourist father, teaching his baby son how to walk, inadvertently stepped out onto the bike path right before me. Though my GPS watch later showed I was doing a mere 5 miles an hour, I still didn't have time to react.

In a split second I had a choice.

Hit the baby?

Or hit the deck?

No one hits a baby.

I somehow (through the grace of God) managed to throw myself up and backward—a move that would have made an Olympic high-jumper proud.

As I went through the air, I wondered if I'd still be able to do my cross-country skate.

Then as I landed with a dull concussive THUD, I had my answer.

I was broken, and badly. But the baby and dad were all right.

The words of Dr. Dyer resonated through my head, "Everything happens for a reason."

I wiggled my fingers, then my toes, then looked at the father, the boy, and the sun shining above. Life is good. I thought. Life is good.

And then, as I lay on the ground like a splayed, broken chicken, I grabbed my left leg, held my breath, and pulled it over to my right. This move likely saved my life. It turns out shards of my femur were less than a centimeter from my femoral artery. Had I moved wrong, or perhaps left my leg in that position, I would have bled to death.

With that done, I began to smile.

I knew something amazingly positive would come out of this experience—and had to—if I were to survive.

I was lucky to be alive, and it still took someone else's blood coursing through my veins to keep me going.

Doctors didn't know if they could put my leg back together. But I knew something amazing would come of this experience.

And something did.

Though I now have a titanium femur and hip, and I've had a total of 10 knee operations and no left ACL, and despite being told I had the "world's flattest (and worst) feet" by podiatrist after podiatrist, I now run barefoot 10 to 20 miles a day.

Doctors said I'd never be able to run again, that I'd be lucky to keep my leg, and lucky to walk. But it was only by feeling the ground, by connecting to the earth, that I was able to heal, get balanced, and run again, despite one leg being shorter than the other.

I've been a professional athlete and coach for the better part of 20 years, just not in the barefoot running world. However, with the inspiration of Jessica Lee, I now coach, write, and speak before others about barefoot running, healing, and connecting to the earth.

I know I was given a second lease on life, and a chance to help others.

"Everything happens for a reason."

From Broken to Barefoot

After finding a way out of a rehab hospital, I ventured into nature to heal. At first, I could crutch only a few hundred yards, alternating deep breathing and meditation to block the pain. But then, over time, my body relaxed and began to grow stronger.

I went from a few hundred yards, to a few miles. I even crutched the Bolder Boulder 10K, and then the Denver Half-Marathon. I wanted to demonstrate how much we can accomplish if we believe in ourselves, no matter what.

From there I continued to spend more time in nature, crutching each morning before the sunrise, and then back again at dusk. I found something special at these times of the day, something sacred in the silence.

Being forced to go slow, I began viewing the world in a different way too. I was seeing things differently, more vividly, and with vibrant color. One morning I stopped to stare at the dewdrop on a leaf, just as the sun began to rise. I began to see all the colors of the rainbow in that drop. It inspired me, and I began to cry. I soon began carrying my camera and capturing amazing healing pictures both at sunrise and sunset. They're now available at galleries around the world.

And I continued to heal. I went from crutching, to walking, and then to jogging. Trouble was, once I tried running, my body began to fall apart. With a nearly 1-inch leg length discrepancy, I couldn't get balanced, no matter how much I tried. I went from one overuse injury to another.

It was frustrating, being out on the trails, or out on the roads, stopping to modify my insoles or orthotics on the fly, stuffing another heel wedge here, or trimming more cork there. Having worked with custom insoles and orthotics in the past, I was a walking insole modification shop. And yet I couldn't get it right.

I wanted to scream out in profanity, or just to cry on the trails. Why couldn't I run pain-free?

I saw doctors, physical therapists, chiropractors, and acupuncturists who all said the same thing, "You'll never run again."

I just couldn't believe it. I wouldn't. There had to be a way. What I needed was a dynamic super-computer that could change or modify my insoles on the fly, depending on the terrain and condition of my feet.

And then one day, I accidentally stumbled upon the solution. As I was struggling on a hot summer's "run," future Olympic champion Constantina Diță, training in Boulder's high altitude, flew by me with a smile. I so desperately wanted to run like her: smiling, effortlessly, and without suffering. In agony, I was frustrated and out of ideas. I didn't even know how to get home without more grisly pain. And so, I took off my shoes, and limped home.

It was the best thing I ever could have done.

At home I looked up more cures for ailing feet, this time Morton's toe. Maybe I had Morton's toe and it was the cause of my problems. But on a Google search, I stumbled across an article by orthopedic surgeon Dr. Joseph Froncioni entitled, "Athletic Footwear and Running Injuries: Essay on the Harmful Effects of Modern Running Shoes." Since I'd just walked home barefoot, I decided to read the article. My jaw hit the floor.

Fewer injuries in less expensive shoes than in more expensive ones. Higher impact in a shoe than out. Perceived safety of cushioning actually harms feet. Better balance and control in thinner, less cushioned shoes. Children in third-world countries are far less likely to have fallen arches and foot problems. The insights went on and on.

And so, two days later, I decided to give it a try. After all, I was already broken. What did I have to lose?

You'd think as a professional athlete I would have tried to see how far I could go barefoot. But I didn't. Instead, as "Mr. Plantar Fasciitis" (I was known for acute plantar fasciitis just by walking across my living room floor without my custom orthotics and motion control shoes), I went out and jogged 100 yards on the local bike path. Then I walked home, grabbing the ground with my toes, trying to strengthen my arches.

And then I iced, for two days straight.

On the third day I went out again. This time a bit farther, 200 yards. And then again, I iced.

Two days later I repeated, 300 yards. Then 400 yards.

Going out every other day I began to get stronger and stronger.

Within three months I'd adapted on the roads, running 10K's and fast, faster than I ever had in a shoe. And that was just the beginning. Now I'm running barefoot on trails, gravel, snow, hot melting asphalt and more. I run 10 to 20 miles a day without shoes, and love running uphills, if not mountains, grabbing with my toes and bounding along. I'm even known to chase a cyclist or two on the road.

How did I do this despite being barefoot? Because being barefoot wasn't the hindrance. Wearing shoes was. Since I was wearing shoes, I couldn't feel the ground, modulate impact, learn to run light, or get balanced. Once I took off my shoes, my feet began to wake up, to grow strong, and become springs. I became aware and in doing so became light, nimble, and far more efficient. I was no longer running, but dancing on the roads, with nature and with my surroundings.

My perception of the world around me changed too, as I become one with my world, rather than one trying to conquer it. I became more peaceful and quiet, as the incessant chatter of the mind melted away. And my running transformed—from a run to a dance, a dance with nature, a dance with my surroundings, a dance to heal, and a dance of joy.

I was running again, mile after effortless mile, without pain, fast, light, and free!

Life-Altering Benefits of Barefoot Running

This book exists to share what I've learned with you, so that you can also reap the life-altering benefits of barefoot running.

- If you've never run before, this book will be your guide to running with minimal injury and maximum health and joy.

- If you're already a runner, this book will show you a much more satisfying way of getting into the zone and improving your stride, form, and performance.

- If you're overcoming an injury—as I was—this book will explain how barefoot running can strengthen your feet and arches in ways you never dreamed possible.

- And if you're simply craving a more spiritual connection to the world, barefoot running will give you that as well.

- If you aren't ready to plunge fully into barefoot running, this book is still for you, as it explains how you can ease into barefoot running using minimalist shoes—and that some runners do well sticking with such shoes permanently.

Your Step-by-Step Guide

You won't have to tear off your shoes until Chapter 5. First, I want to give you a brief introduction to barefoot running and why it's so darned good for you—even if you are among those who still think it's a preposterous idea but were just curious enough to pick up this book.

These first few chapters discuss why barefoot running is a safer alternative and even more satisfying than running shod. I expand my own story because, despite my flat feet and a titanium rod in my leg, barefoot running saved my athletic career. Imagine what it might do for you.

Of course, new barefoot runners need some of the basics, and that's in the chapters leading up to Chapter 5 as I help you work up to walking on a broad expanse of green grass. We stride right into the warm-up exercises in preparation for a real road trip in chapters 6, 7, and 8.

Not every road is smooth and straight, so I'll show you how to make your feet into "all terrain vehicles" and anticipate the roads less traveled and the unpredictable weather conditions in chapters 10 and 11.

This comprehensive guide would not be complete without a serious discussion of nutrition in Chapter 9. Unfortunately, injuries often come with running—mostly while wearing shoes—but they don't have to be surprises, and surely you will need to know how to overcome any injuries that sideline you because you will want to be back out there quickly. Chapter 12 discusses the proven ways to stay healthy.

Two special populations that are often overlooked in books on running are children and seniors. Their special issues with barefoot running are discussed in chapters 14 and 15.

It seems odd to discuss footwear in a book about running without shoes, but Chapter 16 introduces you to the minimalist footwear that you might want to try first or forever.

Once you've mastered the basics and discovered the joy in running and truly feeling the earth beneath your feet, you may remain barefoot for life.

PART I

Why on Earth Would You Want to Run Barefoot?

*Jogging is very beneficial. It's good for your legs and your feet.
It's also very good for the ground. It makes it feel needed.*
—Charles M. Schulz

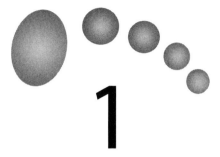

1

Barefoot Running vs. Running in Shoes

If you change the way you look at things, the things you look at change.
—Wayne Dyer

How could something we have for free—our bare feet—be better than something that costs $150?

For many, it seems counterintuitive that running barefoot could be superior to running shod. After all, shoes are designed to protect our feet, and modern running shoes are created by experts working with cutting-edge science and technology to maximize our comfort and safety.

What's seldom mentioned is that these increasingly expensive shoes have done nothing to reduce runner injuries. On the contrary, injuries—to Achilles tendons, tibias, knees, and other essential body parts—have been going up over the years along with shoe prices. Just as surprising was a study that showed runners using shoes costing $95 and up had more than twice as many injuries as those wearing shoes costing $40 or less.

The truth is that running in shoes is high impact, heel-centric, promotes bad form, is relatively unstable and inflexible, tends to weaken rather than strengthen your feet, and dampens your connection to the world around you. In contrast, barefoot running is low-impact, toe-centric, promotes good form, enhances stability and adaptability, strengthens your feet in miraculous ways, and provides delightful sensory and spiritual connections to the earth.

Low-Impact vs. High-Impact Running
(Why the Cheaper Shoes May Be the Best Bargain After All)

Our feet have the most nerve endings of any part of the body, tied only with our hands and genitals. And nerve endings aren't to make us ticklish. They're to help and protect us. So when we run, our feet have a natural desire to "feel" what's going on. It allows them to adjust to different surface conditions on a moment-by-moment basis.

When we wear cushioned shoes, though, it dampens the ability of our feet to sense what's happening beneath them. We'll therefore automatically hit the ground extra hard with each step just to compensate for not feeling the ground directly.

Here's how the problem was explained by orthopedic surgeon Joseph Froncioni in the pivotal article that changed my life:

> During barefoot running, the ball of the foot strikes the ground first and immediately starts sending signals to the spinal cord and brain about the magnitude of impact and shear, getting most of its clues about this from the skin contact with the surface irregularities of the ground. Take away this contact by adding a cushioned substance and you immediately fool the system into underestimating the impact. Add a raised heel and the shod runner is forced to land on it. Strap the cushioning on tightly with the aid of a sophisticated lacing system and you block out shear as well, throwing the shock-absorption system even further into the dark. The system responds by landing harder in an attempt to compress the cushion and "feel" the ground.

Compounding this behavior is the belief propagated by advertising that super-expensive shoes provide super-protection, which leads runners to feel they can strike hard because their shoes are absorbing the impact. A study in *Nature* estimated a runner will strike the ground 2 to 3 times harder with shoes than without them, which helps explain why expensive shoes cause a higher percentage of injuries than the less-cushioned shoes purchased at lower cost. The greater the amount of cushioning, the more we automatically compensate by stepping with greater force and the more confident we feel that striking hard will do no harm.

In fact, though, the repeated high impact creates terrible stress on our ankles, knees, legs, and hips. The cumulative effect of these micro-traumas to which we subject our bodies leads to stress fractures, plantar fasciitis, and a variety of other ailments that sideline as many as two-thirds of runners each year.

Toe vs. Heel Running
(How to Harness the Greatest Marvel of the Human Body)

When we run barefoot and with proper form, we land on the balls of our toes. This dissipates the force of each step through our ligaments, tendons, and musculature. The 28 bones in our feet work in harmony with our muscles to absorb shock and bounce back. This giant "spring" is one of the greatest marvels of the human body.

Running shoes, however, typically include heavily cushioned heels. This leads our brains to think, "land heel first, it's safest." The opposite is true. The calcaneous or heel bone is magnificently designed for walking, helping us balance over any kind of terrain, but while running, our bodies are designed to disengage the heel. When we don't, we lose the natural "spring" created from toe running.

Landing on our heels instead sends the shock of the impact straight through to our ankles, knees, hips, back, and neck. It's as if we're striking bone on bone; once the shock travels past the shoe, there's nothing to stop it or absorb the impact.

Natural (Light) Form vs. Poor Form Running
(How to Tell the Smart Runners from the Heavy-Footed Runners)

Babies run barefoot all the time. They move on sprightly tippy-toes, always leaning forward, letting gravity do the work. Then put that baby in shoes. Watch what happens. The baby suddenly becomes the spawn of Frankenstein, taking awkward robotic steps, landing hard, and teetering to stay upright.

What happened to the light, nimble toe dancing?

It disappeared because the shoes locked the baby's feet into awkward positions—and locked out the baby's natural stride.

●°°₀ FOOT NOTE

Feel the ground, feel your form.

Feel the ground, find your stride.

When you feel the ground, you unlock the hidden potential within. Wearing shoes demolishes that process. It's not impossible to have good form with shoes on, but it's harder and requires a lot more conscious effort.

In his bestselling book *Born to Run*, Christopher McDougall talks about running light. This is an essential skill for barefoot running. When we run light, we put less pressure on our joints and muscles, which allows us to run easier, longer, and with fewer injuries.

Indeed, a way to identify which runners have good form is to simply close your eyes and listen.

At a recent clinic at New York's Central Park, we stopped on the path to hear runnings jogging by. We could pick out runners with poor form because we heard them coming from a block away: Clomp! Clomp! Clomp! with their heavily-cushioned shoes striking hard, heel first, onto the paved ground.

The runners with the best form, however, barely made a sound.

When you go barefoot running, listen to the sound your feet make on impact. The more silent you are, the more likely that you're staying on the balls of your feet … and achieving perfect strides.

When you become skilled at this technique, you'll spook runners as you pass them because they won't hear you coming.

But more importantly, you'll go farther and faster than ever before. Because you're putting less work into raising and lowering your body and less stress on your legs, you can devote more energy to moving forward. Run light and you'll find you can run hour after hour, for mile after mile, floating above the terrain almost effortlessly.

Stable and Adaptable vs. "Blind" Running
(How to Harness the Super-Computer in Your Feet)

Feet have a massive group of nerves packed into them. That's because they're designed to be sensitive enough to feel minute changes in surface conditions and to make moment-by-moment adjustments to keep you continuously balanced and safe.

When you wear running shoes, however, it's like wearing boxing gloves while operating heavy machinery (or putting on a blindfold before crossing the street). While you might survive and accomplish your goals with such handicaps, it's a lot harder to remain safe and to react effectively.

With shoes on, you can't feel the ground, so your feet are deprived of the detailed moment-by-moment information they crave. Instead they're sliding around in your shoes, which interferes with balance, and hitting the ground extra hard in an attempt to gather the information they're blocked from obtaining directly through touch. Furthermore, your feet can't grab or move freely within the shoes, and so are substantially limited in the adjustments they can make to provide you with optimal balance and stride.

You might even find yourself curling your toes within your shoes—which is a natural reaction to what's happening within an unnatural environment. Running in shoes gnarls the toes, as there's no room for them to move, and awkward, unnatural movements over time can lead to medical ailments such as hammer toe in which the toes lose flexibility, swell at the joints, and become permanently bent like little hammers pointed toward the ground. Who wants that?

When I was struggling day after day with orthotics and pain, I dreamed of a super-computer that could instantaneously work with my feet. I imagined it adjusting my left orthotic one way, while simultaneously tilting the right one another way. Then a moment later lowering the heel of one foot because it suddenly needed a little more stability, and raising the other to compensate. This super-computer continued to make such micro-adjustments on a moment-by-moment basis to accommodate every tiny change in both my feet and surfaces.

What I desired was something smart and dynamic enough to handle continually different terrain and an always-changing body, so that no matter how strained, sore, or fatigued I became, my orthotics and shoes could adapt in an instant.

Thankfully, I came to realize that what I needed weren't smarter shoes at all. Instead, I simply needed to stop muzzling the super-computer I was born with: the neurological biofeedback mechanism that goes from the acute senses at the bottom of my feet up through my brain, and back again.

There's a reason our feet have been made so super-sensitive, and it's not for tickling. It's to read the ground and make changes on the fly. You can turn on your own incredible, built-in super-computer by taking off your shoes.

Barefoot vs. Shod Running for Children
(Have We Learned Anything from the Ancient Art of Chinese Foot Binding?)

The longer children are barefoot, the greater are their chances of developing powerful, healthy feet with strong arches; and of their mastering balance, enduring impact, and achieving great form. A 1992 study of 2,300 Indian children found that the chances of developing flat feet were over 3 times greater for the kids wearing shoes than for those going bare.

Certainly we abhor the ancient Chinese practice of foot binding. But it's possible that putting shoes on our children, as soon as they can stand, might be a bad parenting choice too. When it comes to shaping the foot, consider the findings of Dr. Bernhard Zipfel and Professor Lee Berger: "Studies of Asian populations whose feet were habitually either unshod, in thong-type sandals, or encased in non-constrictive coverings have shown increased forefoot widths when compared to those of shod populations." So shoes may not only weaken feet but increase the chances of deforming them. A healthy foot, as described later, grows wider to accommodate the forces of running and walking.

Parenting is a series of judgment calls, and choices aren't always clear-cut. For example, if you live near dangerous surfaces that might cut or infect an unwary child, shoes may offer the best protection for your kids. That said, don't make shoes the automatic or default choice. Except for those times when there are strong reasons to wear shoes, seriously consider letting your kids go barefoot.

Barefoot vs. Shod Running for the Elderly
(Why Grandma Needs to Take Off Her Shoes to Stand Tall)

Even if I've convinced you that running bare is good for kids and adults, you may wonder whether it makes sense for older people, but at this point, you can guess my answer. When we get old, we often lose our sense of balance. In fact, one of the major sources of injury and death among the elderly is falling. Going without shoes—an idea that many older people find insane—just might give them a new sense of their natural balance and allay any fears of falling. But it's tough to convince grandma.

Barefoot running, barefoot jogging, and even barefoot walking will help reactivate the senses in an elderly person's feet and restore the natural balance with which we're born—and that shoes disrupt. Feeling the ground will also strengthen the feet, eventually resulting in greater bone density (an ongoing issue for old bones ravaged by osteoporosis), leg strength, core strength, and stability.

In addition, the stimulation of going barefoot will increase an older person's desire to exercise. And there's no better medicine for old age than regular exercise, as it helps avoid becoming bent and brittle and risking fractures, and staves off such killers as heart disease and countless other maladies. The path to going barefoot must be a slow, gradual process, and that's especially critical for the elderly. But with patience, it can add additional years to an already long life.

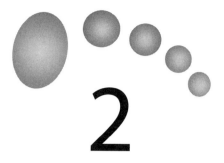

2

Get Grounded by Learning to Play (Again)

The foot feels the foot when it feels the ground.
—Buddha

We all yearn to reconnect with nature. This is visible in our art, entertainment, language, and prayers. In almost all that we do, on some level, we yearn to plug back in.

Throughout the history of mankind, for as long as there've been paintings, drawings, and petroglyphs, humans have been fascinated with nature. We desire to live in the mountains or down by the sea. We put lakes and parks in our cities and bring nature into our homes with aquariums and plants. We use flowers to express love. We paint landscapes, we shoot panoramas, and baseball, our national pastime, takes place on a "field of dreams."

As kids, we yearned to be outdoors. Sadly, there's an epidemic of kids disconnected from nature. Richard Louv, author of *Last Child in the Woods*, says today's children have what he calls "nature deficit disorder." They've been cut off from nature and lost their chance to play outdoors and to connect or plug-in with the world around them.

It's why we're found at the beach on weekends, or in the country, or skiing on the slopes, or craving almost any other activity you can think of. In fact, even when we're indoors watching a movie, chances are nature or a beautiful backdrop is featured prominently throughout the film.

For many, connecting with nature is what draws you to running—and to this book. You yearn to breathe fresh air, quiet the mind, and to be outside—laughing, playing, and enjoying nature, as you once did as a child.

We've almost all become unplugged today. Too much work, too many computers, cell phones, and too many people crammed into high rises and out on the streets. We're slaves to our lives, jobs, and furnishings. It seems there's no end to the commitments, no time to breathe, and no time to be ourselves. And even when we do get outside, we often still feel disconnected—as if there's something missing. It's why we run with our iPods, or our cell phones, or any other distraction we can get our hands on.

Something's missing. Something vital.

Recently, I saw a painting in a coffee shop, titled *Sensual Stroll*. It was a picture of a woman dancing barefoot through the grass. Why is it sensual? Because of the feelings and emotions evoked from being barefoot in the grass.

On the beach, we let our feet squish through the sand and feel the water lap our toes. In the parks, if we're lucky, we take off our shoes and also dance through the grass.

These sensual experiences hearken back to simpler times, to times as a child when we ran free without our shoes, until our parents made us put them on. Maybe learning to tie our shoes wasn't such a good thing after all. It meant we had to wear them. Or, as Danny Dreyer, author of *ChiRunning*, describes in his Foreword to this book, putting on shoes signaled the end of summer's carefree barefoot days, a pair of squeaky new tie-shoes, and the beginning of another year of grade school.

An Inch of Rubber Away from Nirvana

What's missing today is a physical connection to the earth. We're spending too much time indoors, and, even when we're outside for a run, we're separated by an inch of rubber, which is a fantastic resistor to electricity.

This brings us to the physics of getting grounded—how we're truly connected to the earth and vibrate at the same frequency of the earth, what that means to our health, and how barefoot running can help: sensually, physically, and spiritually.

On a spiritual level, we're no longer connected to the ground from where we evolved. On a physical level, we're no longer connected to the earth's magnetic fields and particle charges. On a mental level, we see ourselves as distinctly separate from nature and other living beings.

Since the beginning, we've been in nature, not just foraging for food, not just to survive, but for our enjoyment and spiritual experiences as well. Organized religions give us scenes of Jesus in nature throughout the Bible and images of Buddha on his travels and path toward enlightenment. I contend that we've forgotten who we are spiritually.

Though in many ways we're more advanced than at any other time, we're also the most unplugged. We all feel a desire to connect, to feel the earth and get grounded again. We just have a hard time finding the way or letting ourselves do it.

Perhaps what's missing is that we're no longer touching the ground—literally this time. It's considered dirty, taboo, or even dangerous. As an advanced society, we're told we no longer touch the earth in that way, and we've developed devices (shoes) to keep us above the ground.

As a species we were raised to hunt, farm, gather, and be outdoors. We never evolved to be indoors all day or to wear shoes. We have beautiful strong feet and an incredible means for connecting with nature.

At our barefoot running clinics, it's nothing but ear-to-ear grins once participants shed their shoes and frolic in the grass. It's not just physical; it's soothing on an emotional and spiritual level.

Nature's Drugstore

Disease or its derivative *dis*-ease, comes from an unsettled mind. Connecting with the earth, plugging back in, quiets our minds. Spiritual author Deepak Chopra often describes disease as coming from stress and harmful chemicals (such as cortisol or stress hormones) ravaging our body.

Yet our mind may be the greatest drugstore on earth. We often don't know how a drug works, but know that it triggers the release of chemicals from the brain. When we're grounded and having fun, even a simple smile can produce more powerful cancer-fighting and health-generating drugs than anything else in the world. Perhaps this is a great benefit of barefoot running—connecting with the earth and taking those deep breaths helps heal and center us from deep within.

Getting in Sync

My dogs Pumpkin and Sawa want their food at exactly the same time every day. But how do they know it's time to eat? They're not wearing puppy watches, but their internal clock tells them when to wake, sleep, and even salivate for food. All animals except for humans with our artificial light, computer screens, and TVs have synchronized their body clocks with that of the earth.

By exercising regularly, particularly barefoot and feeling the ground, we can reconnect with and reset our internal clocks.

Reset your clock by getting outside barefooted, preferably at sunrise or sunset, each day. Curl your toes in the dirt, feel the grass, or scrunch along the pavement. I'd recommend walking or running outside on a routine, repetitive basis, particularly at sunrise and sunset, which tends to synchronize our bodies to the 24-hour cycle of the sun. Whatever hour of day you choose, try to go out everyday at that same time.

The body will learn when to rise and when to sleep, when to think, and when to go quiet. This body knowledge helps us let go, relax, and get in sync with the earth.

Spiritual Grounding—Plugging into Source

Although you don't need to be religious or spiritual to enjoy barefoot running, you may find the act of shedding your shoes and touching the ground to be a spiritual experience.

The nomenclature of spirituality isn't what's important. Call it *God, Mother Nature, Universe, Chi, Love, Source,* or whatever term best fits your belief system, but the universal power is all around us and supports us with life-giving energy. To me, touching the earth helps me plug back into Source. I tap into this life force and seem to be magically revitalized.

It's as if while wearing shoes or being indoors all day, we become unplugged from an energy source, and when we're barefoot and outdoors, we're plugged back in when our feet touch the earth. If only we could run cars on that energy, we'd have the world energy crisis solved.

The physics of getting grounded

Getting grounded isn't merely a spiritual feeling; it's literally "grounded" in physics.

Since the beginning of time, we humans have walked, slept, and spent most of our time with our bare feet on the ground, unaware that this physical contact transfers natural healing electrical energy to our bodies.

During the past 50 years or so, for the first time in history, our modern lifestyle has disconnected us from the earth's energy making us more vulnerable to stress and illness. We wear insulating rubber or synthetic-soled shoes, travel around in metal boxes with rubber wheels, and eat, sleep, and work in structures raised above the ground. New research is showing that when we reconnect to the earth by way of our bare feet, or by using a grounding device, a myriad of things happen to support health and vitality.

First, the earth immediately equalizes your body to the same energy level, or potential, as the earth, synchronizing your internal biological clock, hormonal cycles (like cortisol), and physiological rhythms. People who have used devices designed to maintain their connection with the surface of the earth when they sleep report that they sleep better, have less pain and stress, and recover faster from trauma.

Second, when you reconnect to the negatively charged electrons on the surface of the earth, the build-up of positively charged free radicals in your body that leads to inflammation is neutralized. Chronic inflammation has been implicated in all types of serious health issues including diabetes, Alzheimer's, cancer, leukemia, heart disease, and autoimmune disorders such as rheumatoid arthritis, multiple sclerosis, and many others. When research subjects were connected to the earth, medical thermal images showed decreased inflammation in only minutes.

Third, the human body carries an electrical charge and is swimming in a field of electricity. When you connect to the earth, you can dissipate the electrical charge caused by a build-up of your body's own electricity, and you are protecting yourself from the stressful electro-magnetic fields all around us. These may be harmful to both your physiology and psychology (and are particularly harmful to developing children).

No matter where you are on the earth (some places less than others), you're constantly bombarded by these electro-magnetic waves. New studies and products continually address this issue, which some call "electro-pollution" or "geopathic" stress, referring to the geo-magnetic relationship between us as biological creatures and the geo-magnetically charged earth.

We've all had the experience of being shocked by static electricity. Recently, Jessie and I traveled the aisles of the local supermarket, being zapped by each other aisle after aisle. We carry a charge, and this charge builds up as we swim in a sea of electro-pollution from cell phones, cordless phones, electrical cords and wires, microwaves, refrigerators, and more. In our modern environments, unless we're in direct contact with the earth, we're carrying an extra electrical charge with our bodies throughout the day.

Unfortunately, as cell phone use becomes more ubiquitous, electro-pollution continues to rise, as do corresponding health risks. We're not even safe in our beds at home; we're still bombarded by electrical radiation as we sleep, from cell phone signals, household appliances, the wiring in the wall behind our beds, and even microwave towers miles down the street.

It turns out that the earth has a frequency, or a heartbeat, called the Schumann Resonance, of approximately 7.83 hertz. This number is important because it's the same frequency our brains use to survive and thrive. In other words, our vibrations are matched or we vibrate at the same frequency of the earth. Put another way, we evolved in sync with the frequency or heartbeat of the earth.

NASA scientists have known this for years. In early space missions, astronauts became surprisingly weak and ill when they went into space and left the resonance of the earth behind. They now alleviate this distress by having a vibrational device attached to the ships that resonates at the Schumann Resonance—by matching to the frequency of the earth, spacecraft help astronauts stay in sync.

(According to an NIH report, "The Schumann Resonance signal provides a brain frequency range matching electromagnetic signal, providing the synchronization needed for intelligence.")

We vibrate in sync with the world around us. When our environment is out of sync, we're out of sync too, which can have significant harmful effects on our bodies and minds. Studies are showing that when our environment is not vibrating around 7.83 hertz, for instance, in an environment bombarded by cell phone radiation or other electrical appliances, brain wave function can be disturbed (causing ADD-like symptoms, depression, and other psychological conditions) along with medical conditions affected by electrical charges.

While the earth's frequency averages 7.83 Hz, it cycles throughout the day, peaking twice both around 8 a.m. and 5 p.m. These peaks help keep our bodies in tune with the 24-hour cycle of the planet. Since our bodies and minds are in tune with the earth, these cycles give us our circadian rhythm or internal 24-hour clock, helping us naturally know when to rise and when to sleep. However, when our environment's overloaded with charges, and we're surrounded by electrical devices, we're thrown out of sync with this natural circadian rhythm.

Being barefoot for just a few minutes a day may not be enough to bring you back in sync. It's not just a matter of dissipating the charges, but of re-synchronizing ourselves with the cycle and vibration of the earth. This takes time, such as long barefoot walks, runs, or hikes daily or twice daily (following the cycles of the earth).

Additionally, being barefoot for a few minutes each day doesn't protect us from the harmful electromagnetic frequencies we're virtually swimming in. To protect ourselves, we must be grounded. When we connect to the earth, we become part of the earth's circuit. We not only begin vibrating with the earth, but it helps protect us and keep charges from entering our bodies.

If you've ever heard of lightning striking a car, the reason people aren't killed isn't because of the thin rubber tires. It's because the electricity travels around the car instead of into it, and then exits through the ground. This is called the Farridy Cage effect. Our skin works the same when we're connected to the ground. Electrical waves hit our skin and go around our bodies to the ground when we're barefoot. In this way, grounding protects us from the incredibly harmful electromagnetic pollution. The more time you spend being grounded each day, the better.

This is why products such as grounding sheets and grounding pads have come about. Like going barefoot, these products help in 3 key ways. First, they help us shed excess ions and reduce free radicals. Second, they help sync us with the earth while we sleep. Third, they help protect us from the sea of electromagnetic pollution.

Grounding sheets and pads, such as those from Barefoot Health, Inc. (www.barefoothealth.com), have a silver or carbon mesh and plug directly into the ground via a wire and grounding rod or into a properly grounded electrical outlet. You can sleep on them, lay them on your office chair, or even on your favorite couch. Others like me use them at their work desks and swear by them for increased productivity, improved health (greater cold resistance), and far less stress at work, even while bombarded by high levels of EMFs.

Earth conductive bed sheets were even used by Lance Armstrong's Tour de France team. The sheets helped athletes reduce inflammation, prevent tendonitis, accelerate recovery and wound healing, and improve the quality of sleep. By being literally grounded and plugged in to the earth, the athletes recovered faster and improved performance. This is no small matter in one of the most severe tests of endurance on the planet.

But you don't need to be a professional athlete to benefit from improved sleep, better recovery, and less pain. By reconnecting to the earth you'll feel better, recover faster, and sleep better.

Stepping Off the Cliff

Jessica once asked me, "How did you *know* you'd be okay going barefoot?" It's a great question, but somehow I just *knew* this was the path for me.

While I'd only read a few online articles about barefoot running before my first forays sans shoes, it made perfect sense. In my meditations, I heard, *You've tried everything else. Why not give running barefoot a try?* When I began, I called it the grand-experiment with little idea of where it would take me. But with every fiber in my being I knew the experiment would be a success.

Perhaps we can do anything we believe we can. Perhaps someday we'll all walk on water, or fly above the seas unassisted. Believing is extraordinarily powerful. It's how I rode across the country, 5,000 miles in 40 days, solo and unsupported, because I knew in my heart I could make it. What could we do if we always listened to that little voice that *knows* we can accomplish things?

I had no fear of barefoot running. Why? Because I was already in pain and told I'd never be able to run again. It was the same tune I heard as an 11-year-old when I was told that without my ACL (anterior cruciate ligament) I'd never be able to run or play again like the other kids. The doctors were wrong, and I learned an extremely important lesson. I learned that I was in greater charge of my health and destiny than anyone else—even the so-called experts.

So decades later as an adult, being told (twice now) that I could never run again was the best news I could ever hear. It liberated me to take risks and think outside the box. Of course, in my mind barefoot running was the least risky endeavor of all. The bigger risk would have been giving up running and letting my body gradually wither away. To me, the risk of a barefoot-induced injury paled in comparison to the disease and illness that would set in with a sedentary lifestyle.

I knew there was a way to heal and run again, a way that was simple, true, and easy. I just had to find it. But it was closer than I ever thought. I'd seen it in my meditations—myself running along effortlessly without shoes. At first, I saw it as a metaphor, not as a model. But what better solution than the most natural one of them all? After all, we're all born barefoot. Where's the risk? We certainly wouldn't have told cavemen to stay indoors for lack of clean trails, clear paths, and protective shoes.

And so I had faith, stepped off the cliff into the unknown, and there I found my true nature.

And you can, too. Take off those shoes, believe you can do it, know you can do it, and find the new you. How often do we get to reinvent and rediscover something about ourselves? This is an amazing chance for self-discovery and greater awareness. Just believe in yourself, in the power of your feet, envision yourself barefoot, and step out into a brave new world.

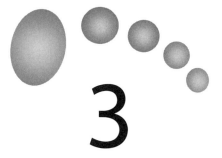

3

Humanplay: Dancing with Nature

Man is most nearly himself when he achieves the seriousness of a child at play.
—Heraclitus

Once barefoot, we're no longer simply running. We're now dancing through the woods, on the trails, and wherever we go. We land light, feel the ground, look around, then spring off the next foot, as nimble as the animals that live out in nature. We're hopping from rock to rock and step to step. It's more than child's play. I call it *humanplay*, or doing what nature intended us to do.

Running in the Now

For me, barefoot running is an exercise in mindful meditation. I can clear out my mind and let go of thought. I become keenly aware of what I'm doing and everything around me, but not of the incessant inner chatter. Being mindful or present of each step, there's no worrying about the past, no concern for the future. I'm simply living each present moment, with each and every step.

Once you start, you begin looking around and seeing the world in a different way. You leave your troubles behind and focus on the feeling of your feet on the ground and the movement of your body. If you're thinking about the past or the future, you can't take stock of your condition. You can't hear your footfalls, feel the terrain change, or know anything going on around you. If you're dwelling on a problem, or focusing on the future, you may be completely unaware of the glass bottle shards coming your way.

Letting go of your over-abundance of thought leaves you free to explore and truly experience your true nature and the world all around you. You smell, hear, see, and sense things you've never noticed before. You notice the birds, sky, trees, and everything around as if it were your first time.

Running in the now, in complete awareness, you feel the surreal sensation of floating along. You hear the sound of the birds or the wind swirling between trees or even buildings. You feel the warm glow of the sun's early blanket on your arms or even the powerful, healing whoosh of your own breath, drawn in and out.

Running Awarefoot

Running barefoot means running aware.

When you're barefoot, you have to know what's in front of you and where to step. You need to know the temperature, conditions, and many other factors around you. And you must know your internal conditions—those of muscles, joints, ligaments, and tendons along with your fatigue levels, fluid levels, and especially your mental state.

To avoid the pebble, rock, or shard of glass, you are not necessarily scanning the ground ahead of you with eyes cast downward—ever vigilant for a discarded, broken beer bottle or jagged rock. Instead, you must open your mind and your awareness by shutting off your thoughts and becoming, as I like to say, "awarefoot." Simply feel the ground, feel your breaths, and then open up your senses, yet without thought.

Once you connect to the ground, and open up your mind, a whole world of awareness instantly beckons—even that hazardous twisted soda can and its potential to send you to the ER for stitches. Animals feel the ground and are connected to the earth and their surroundings. Plugged in and free from extraneous thought, they're constantly living in the now, aware of everything around and underfoot. It's a living awareness of the earth and their surroundings that allows them to avoid storms, forest fires, and tsunamis.

We humans too have built-in awareness. For example, we manage to instantly turn our cars without thought, swerving just at the last second, to avoid a collision. Our hair stands on end if we sense danger in a dark alley. But we wouldn't tap into this sixth sense if a CD was blaring in the car or the iPod was cranked up.

So too our senses can be dulled by that inch of rubber between us and the ground.

By cultivating our awareness by touching the ground and opening our minds, we improve every aspect of our lives. We go from simply living or being, letting the world carry us along, unaware and oblivious of our surroundings, to being fully aware and awake.

Become the Observer

I remember how loud and clear my inner voice was to me on my solo 5,000-mile bike ride across the country. During interviews I'd end up saying, "We rode 200 miles today," or "No matter what, we'll make it there."

To this, the keen interviewer always asked, "*We*? Don't you mean *you*? I thought you were alone?"

And to this I'd respond, "Yes, I was alone. But there was 'me' the person on the bicycle, and the infinite observer, that voice in my head that was cheering me along."

To me, the observer, or what I call the infinite observer is that quiet inner voice, watching the action yet remaining neutral to it all. It's the one cheering you on as you get into barefoot running, the voice that helps keep you from doing too much. It's the still, small voice that's always with you, if you can take the time to quiet your mind and listen.

When you expand your awareness by running barefoot, you expand your mind. You become the observer rather than just another participant. This enables you to let go of judgment and experience the world more fully, taking joy in everything you hear, feel, see, touch, taste, or sense.

For instance, when you're the observer, even if you do too much and need to take time to heal, you're not upset, instead you learn from the experience, enjoy the time off, and enjoy every step of the process. There's no longer a good or bad experience, nor a right or wrong decision. Things stop being judged and simply become experiences that enrich our lives and help us to grow. By being the observer of our experiences, rather than being trapped by them, we become truly free. Free to let go, free to make changes, free to experience, run barefoot, and to grow.

When you are the infinite observer, the one aware of the entire world around you, you become a true player in the game of life, and a rule-maker too. You can make your character be whoever you wish him or her to be. You can be or do anything you desire. You can change roles at the drop of a hat, and you can change your life.

By changing your awareness, you change your very existence along with the world you live in. Your world expands far beyond the reaches of your walls and the rubber of your shoes. You see yourself from new perspectives and vantage points, both inside and outside of yourself. As your perspective changes, your entire mindset changes.

When you begin to become truly aware, an exercise you can cultivate through meditation and running barefoot, a veil lifts and you start to see what's on the inside. And that's where the special journey truly begins. At first, your awareness goes to your external senses—what you're seeing, touching, tasting, hearing, and smelling (not to mention what you're running on and where to step). Next it goes to your internal environment, how you're feeling physically on the inside. But then it goes somewhere truly special into the stillness or what I call the infinite. What do I hear in that still, small voice? What's in the silence and infinity of my mind? What is there when there are no sounds, no chatter, or no inner voice? What does it mean to connect to all and to feel truly alive?

You can begin to cultivate your awareness, to expand your consciousness, and to sense what's inside, outside, and all around—all by beginning to walk or run barefoot.

Exercise: Warm up Your Awareness

Try this: For this exercise, you can do either a barefoot walk or barefoot run. It's also fun to do with a friend, sharing your experiences as you go along.

See: Head out on a familiar road, trail, or anywhere you desire. Take stock of your surroundings by asking yourself what you see around you. Take it all in, from the trail before you, to the plants and leaves on the trees, even the bugs and the dirt. Leave no sight untouched, from the smallest, to the most distant, even the faintest of glows.

Hear: Next ask what you hear, stretch your senses, and listen for new sounds. Perhaps at first you only hear footfalls, then a distant plane, far away conversations, birds or more. Can you hear the crickets or the wind rustling—sounds you've missed before? Notice how new noises come into play as your awareness warms up through this exercise. Challenge yourself and ask, *Can I hear anything else? What can I hear in the "silence"?*

Taste: After hearing, what do you taste? Is it sweat, saliva, or blood? Perhaps the metal caps on your teeth, the salt from food you just ate, or something else? What new awareness can you awaken?

Smell: Next what do you smell? Is it the woods? The trees? An animal? Person? Your sweat or something else? Keep smelling the world all around you. Try and take it in and sense all that you can. (An ancient animal tracking trick I like is to curl your tongue back to the roof of your mouth and breathe the air in through your nose. Can you smell anything new this way?)

Feel: Now what do you feel around you? Can you sense the ground? The sun's warmth on your arms? The energy of people, animals, buildings, or trees all around? Try to feel everything you can. Watch as your awareness expands. This is where being barefoot particularly comes into play. Can you feel the pebbles? The stones? The warmth or coolness of the ground? The energy from the earth? The cracks in the pavement? The way your foot hits the ground or pulls at the earth? Can you feel your muscles tightening as you connect? Can you feel how erect you're standing? Your core? How you're carrying your shoulders, your head, and everything in your body?

Now that you've taken stock of the world all around, it's time to go to the most special place of all—the world of the inside. What do you feel on the inside, not in your body, but in the silence?

Go beyond your mind and listen to the silence. What do you hear now?

Feel, Focus, Finesse

Being aware is much more than just feeling the ground. It's feeling your entire body at work and at play. It's making adjustments with the feet and the legs, and it's feeling and tinkering with your body to see what works best.

Next time you switch on a NASCAR race, observe the race car drivers on a hot lap, trying to nurse the fastest time out of their cars. Do you think they're on the com line with the pit or relaxing with an extra-cushioned seat? Not a chance. They need to be fully aware and sensing everything. So they have an extra stiff seat, a firm, yet relaxed grip on the wheel, and ultra-thin shoes, which allow them to feel the cars' vibrations, the undulation of the track, and every sensation imaginable. It's not about brute force in a race car; it's about feel, focus, and finesse.

For runners, feel, focus, and finesse means sensing the terrain and everything our body does. We need to sense it all, then let go of it all. If not, we'd have information overload; for a race car driver that'd mean a nasty or deadly crash. For us, it could lead to a trip, fall, or injury. Instead we must be aware, and then let go. Remaining focused yet relaxed helps us flow with the terrain, letting our feet guide us on cruise-control. That's why being aware and emptying the mind are so important.

When you're barefoot, you feel every sensation, every movement of your head, every swing, sway, or twitch in your body all through your feet.

Feel the Ground for Better Balance

Stand up, right now. Now touch your nose while standing on just one leg. Easy. Now close your eyes. Do it again. Did you start teetering? Did you begin to fall? When you lose just one of your senses (in this case, your sight), you're instantly off balance.

That's what running is like when you wear shoes. When you lose one of your senses (the sense of feel), you can't feel the ground. You're running blind and wobbly. I'm surprised we can stay upright at all. Yet when you take off your shoes, your balance instantly improves, and only gets better from there.

By feeling the ground, the impact, and everything going on in our bodies, we learn to change our strides and modulate impact. This makes us the captains of our own destiny. Hit the ground with bare feet, and they feel free and invincible. But they still don't feel the ground fully in minimalist shoes. Without this feedback, nor having strengthened the feet, they can't hear their bodies telling them to stop.

Without shoes, your skin gets sore, your muscles fatigue, and you pay the piper right away. It's hard to say "no pain, no gain" when your stride falls apart, your footfalls go to heck, your feet begin to blister, and the pounding soon begins. Even the strongest ego quickly says *no mas*. Yet with shoes on, even minimalist ones, you lack instant feedback and response. There's no evident reason to stop or slow down. Instead you may go for days or weeks before it's too late. But then, it's not a blister that stops you, but dreaded stress fractures or tendonitis.

Hear the Dirt Beneath Your Feet

Nature's where I've gone for healing, solace, and peace of mind. She's the world's greatest reset button, helping me prioritize, put things in perspective and make them clear once again. Barefoot on a mountain top, in a park, or on a beach, it's hard to harbor worries of the world. Nature's where I go to help quiet my mind and end the incessant inner chatter. Running barefoot, I tread lightly into the silence, hearing nature's secret symphony, and the dirt beneath my feet.

In 1992 while racing bicycles in Europe, I was waved by a race safety official into an oncoming car. I suffered nerve damage to L4 and L5 vertebrae in my lower back after flipping over the hood. For three years, I suffered tremendous back pain and couldn't get various muscles to fire, specifically my glutes and psoas. I visited specialists, pain clinics, chiropractors, and acupuncturists. The medical professionals all came to the same conclusion: the more exercise I did, the greater my pain would be. The prognosis across the board was rest and a lifestyle that no longer involved exercise and fitness.

Yet trail running became my miracle cure. A massage therapist and Pilates instructor's core strengthening and unique foam roll and tennis ball exercises also helped me along my way.

When trail running, my body was forced to balance itself without conscious efforts. Over time my body relearned to fire muscles laid dormant by the accident. I went from slow hiking, to jogging, then running halfway up Pikes Peak Mountain (a 14,000-foot peak in Colorado Springs) 2 to 3 times a week (with 3 dogs, including my trusty dog Pumpkin who is still running with me to this day).

Before trail running, doctors couldn't find any discernible firing of my glutes and psoas muscles (those near the groin that lift the leg). Yet afterward, they worked great, giving birth to a new career in cycling, skating, and long-distance triathlons. In 2003, while training for track cycling, I set a personal record of 1,650-pound repeats on a hip-sled—a weight-lifting machine you power with your glutes. I then went on to get seventh at the masters national championship in cycling, beat the national cycling team in the Olympic Sprints event on the track, and in skating even got a sponsorship from Rollerblade.

Yes, I didn't go on to compete in the Tour de France, but I learned much more, about hanging in there, never giving up, visualizing my muscles working again, having faith, seeing myself heal, and letting nature guide and heal me. I'm convinced it was being out on the trails, on my toes, imbalanced yet perfectly balanced in nature that helped or allowed me to heal.

Healing in Nature

Nature has a healing energy. And running trails, particularly rocky, uneven ones, does more to help us regain our balance and strength than almost anything else. I see so many people going out in nature with poles to balance themselves. While I understand they have them for safety, I believe if they start slowly, and just do a hundred yards at a time without their poles—preferably barefoot, or definitely in minimalist shoes where they can feel the ground—they will do more to regain their balance than almost anything else.

The poles act as crutches metaphorically. Literally, they're like the crutches we use on our feet we call "shoes." Shoes seem like safety devices at the time, supportive devices that give us freedom. But what they do is block the circuit of feedback and energy from the ground to our minds. They block our ability to feel the ground and find balance, and they rob our muscles of the challenge of supporting our own weight. As I found on the trails, even muscles clinically tested that showed zero signs of firing may find a way to fire again.

For me, it was out in nature that got me going again. I was out crutching in nature within 2 weeks of my 2006 accident. I began with only a few hundred yards, but was back out in the healing power of nature. From there I built up to almost twice daily until I healed—and continue this practice every day.

I'm often tromping along a trail barefoot when I freeze in my tracks, jaw dropped at the beauty all around me, and a watercolor sky up above. Often a runner will pass, or perhaps a couple of runners, pushing hard perhaps with iPods blaring, while struggling in their shoes. They may look back with inquisitive gazes, wondering what in the world I'm staring at. Some may even stop and ask, unable to perceive what I see.

While we might move faster wearing shoes over sharp stones or tough branches, if we're rushed and unplugged from our surroundings, is there much difference between a trail run and a treadmill? After all, what's the point? Is it merely to finish the run, raise our heart rates, run in a "zone," or reach our destination? Isn't there something more?

Now I love going fast, and as a racer I appreciate a great pace—flying free and dancing silly while speeding along a road or trail, but not at the expense of missing the moment or truly having fun. To me, they go hand in hand.

In the old days on long runs I slogged along in my shoes, focused on time and heart rate and miles to go, rather than on the beauty all around me. At these times I was oblivious to my surroundings, often tired and miserable, and bored beyond belief. Those runs never seemed to end.

But now, out in the woods, I leave behind the iPod. Watching the sunset, hearing my footfalls, and feeling the ground opens me up to the experience, while leaving me invigorated and at peace. I never feel bored. Instead I'm like a kid again, seeing the world anew. Once barefoot, even the most "boring" trail becomes new and filled with excitement. I am a kid again.

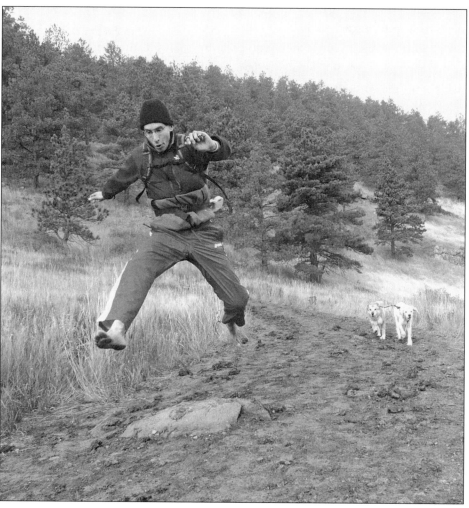

Michael on the trail, flying and feeling like a kid again with Pumpkin and Sawa.

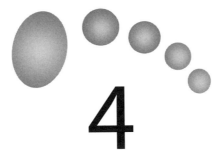

4

Born to Run Barefoot: The Philosophy of an Age-Old Movement

I will always listen to my coaches. But first I listen to my body. If what they tell me suits my body, great. If my body doesn't feel good with what they say, then always my body comes first.

—Haile Gebrselassie

If humans were meant to run barefoot, why would taking off our shoes require a how-to guide?

The fact of the matter is, the vast majority of us who grew up in developed countries didn't grow up barefoot. As a result, the muscles, tendons and ligaments in our feet, ankles, knees, legs, and hips have atrophied or never fully developed. Traditional running shoes have taught us to run with unnatural form in many cases encouraging us to heel strike thus increasing our chance of injury.

This chapter introduces you to the philosophy behind barefoot running, which requires you to make three major shifts in thought:

#1 No pain equals maximum gain.

#2 You must go slow to go fast.

#3 Taking breaks does not mean you are lazy.

Making these paradigm shifts is the best way to transition and ensure a lifetime of happy, injury-free running.

In barefoot running, we're waking up muscles, joints, ligaments, and tendons that have long since been dormant. We're asking muscles to move in ways they're not used to moving; asking joints, ligaments, and tendons to handle forces they have never encountered before; and, to top it off, we're asking our bodies to do all of this new, rather foreign work without support, a safety net, or a cushion that would otherwise be provided by a shoe.

To do this requires growing your own shoes, and they do not grow overnight.

According to Dr. Craig Richards, a researcher at the University of Newcastle in Australia whose article on barefoot running was published in the *British Journal of Sports Medicine*, 6 months is the steepest part of the learning curve for the body, when the most growth and change occur and when you're most susceptible to injury. Richards even suggests, "Muscles used for heel striking have to atrophy to allow for proper form." He believes you make the most significant gains between 6 months and 2 years after you begin barefoot running.

Take it from me, I ran a mere 100 yards barefoot my first day. I then iced for 2 days before running another mere 200 yards. This is how I managed to remain injury-free. Some may run shorter distances to begin. Others may run farther. The key is to let your body dictate how fast, how far, and how often to run.

The second key to staying injury-free is running with natural form. In this chapter, I also address two bones of contention in the running world regarding stride length and foot strike. As a barefoot runner, you'll learn quickly that a forefoot strike will keep you light on your feet, while a heel strike will send you home, and that a shorter, quicker stride is softer and more efficient than a longer stride.

If there are any key points you should take away from this chapter, they're the next three rules. Do your best to commit these to memory.

◐°°°₀ FOOT NOTE

3 Simple Rules for Safety

#1: Stop barefoot running once you stop having fun.

#2: Stop barefoot running once you feel the slightest tweak or twinge of pain.

#3: Never let your pride get in the way of stopping, whether it's to pluck out a pebble wedged into your foot or to put on a minimalist shoe. (Yes, there most certainly are times for wearing shoes. See the chapter on minimalist shoes and other gear.)

Go Slow to Go Fast

Whether you're an elite runner, fast runner, or everyday recreational runner, if you run on a regular basis, expect to slow down as you transition into barefoot running. It's often the fastest runners who are the most challenged when transitioning to barefoot running.

If you're a fast runner, your muscles are strong, but your feet are still weak. This has the potential of getting you into trouble fast. So pay attention to these road signs:

- **Forget Muscle Memory.** You have mile after mile of ingrained habits in your muscle memory. It may be hard to break these habits and get you into proper stride.

- **Change What's Strong.** While many of your muscles are strong, they may not move in the way you need and may even inhibit proper form. For barefoot running you'll need some of your strong muscles (used to carrying a shoe) to relax, and your weak muscles to grow stronger.

- **Slow Down.** If you muscle through on brute strength, you'll tear yourself apart. Many good runners have tried transitioning too quickly without picking up proper form first. This has quickly led to overuse injuries and dreaded stress fractures. The faster you run, the more damage you'll do (and the faster you'll do it) if you head out without proper form. However, it's hard to tell a runner who's been running a 5-, 6-, or 7-minute mile to slow down to a 12- or even a 15-minute mile. Mentally, that's tough, and keeping those reigns on, even tougher.

- **Reawaken Your Feet.** Even if your muscles and skin are strong, and you run with proper form, your sheer mileage can wreak havoc on your feet, calves, and Achilles. Your feet have been locked in a dark box without room to flex, move, or support themselves for years. They need to gradually reawaken. As your skin grows stronger, you strengthen the muscles, tendons, and ligaments and begin to lay down new bone. Bone density increases with stress, but it must do so gradually. Bones will grow stronger by bearing more of the weight (there's no support when barefoot) and by stronger muscles and tendons pulling on the bone. However, if we increase weight bearing too quickly (through mileage) or muscle strength too quickly, we'll tear the bones apart.

Stress fractures are easy to come by while transitioning (and as discussed later, particularly if you don't let your skin be your guide). This is why so many people get stress fractures and tendonitis when starting out in minimalist footwear. They're lots of fun, but if you don't build your feet strong first, and learn to feel the ground, you're in for a world of hurt, no matter how strong you are. In fact, the stronger a runner you are, the harder you may fall.

Be Willing to Start from Scratch

I learned some important lessons along my path to barefoot running.

When I last visited the Newton Shoe Lab in Boulder, Colorado, I met with Danny Abshire, co-founder and inventor of these unique running shoes. He remembered me from visits prior to my getting into barefoot running. At that time I was bruised, battered, frustrated, and dejected. His shoes didn't work. His orthotics didn't work. Nothing seemed to work.

On my recent visit, Danny shared his observations of me from that earlier visit. It wasn't that his shoes didn't work, nor his orthotics. The truth of the matter was I wasn't giving my body time to rest. I was broken, yet I ignored the screams from my body while relentlessly and repeatedly running it into the ground.

Months after graduating from crutches after my accident, I began running, but with lots of pain. Docs said I would never be able to relieve the pain, yet I continued to limp and hobble mile after challenged mile, admittedly at a fast pace when I should have taken it slower. Yet at the time I was still under the delusion that pain equals gain. And so I pushed on, cognizant of the challenges, yet unaware of the solution.

I was desperately trying to find the solution, be it through a cork heel-wedge, a new custom orthotic, an exotic new shoe, or some other complicated combination.

I ignored all practical advice until the day I went barefoot. And Danny reminded me of this.

I had to stop cold, wipe the slate clean, and hit the reset button on my body before I could heal. Only then could I begin rebuilding without carrying my injuries forward.

You may not be "broken" at all. You may even be running stronger than you've ever run before. So this may be a difficult concept to grasp, or you may be saying "not me." It's a mind-bender. But the fastest transition to barefoot running is to slow down and stop. Then rebuild from the ground up. It's the longest solution for the short run, yet the shortest, for the long run.

By starting with a clean slate, you'll let go of nagging injuries, which will allow you to build back faster, stronger, and without old bad habits. At the same time, you'll be preventing blisters, torn muscles, overuse injuries, stress fractures, and more.

The day I went barefoot, I changed my mindset, allowed my body to heal, and was willing to take as many breaks as it took. In short, I let go of a timeline or result and stepped slowly into the unknown.

My skin became my guide and my coach. It was painstakingly slow. But it worked magnificently. By *going slow to go fast*, I slowly worked my way into dancing barefoot within a few short months. By the fourth month, I was running and flying along at subfreezing temperatures chasing cyclists up steep hills. By the sixth month, I could do 10 miles or more. And within my first year, I was turning 20 miles safely, without injury or pain.

Respect Pain

When it comes to pain, I'm a baby. I've also heard Barefoot Ted describe himself the same way. Barefoot Ted is perhaps the most famous barefoot runner in the U.S., in part due to his participation in the "greatest race the world never knew about" chronicled in the book *Born to Run*. This doesn't mean Ted and I are weak runners or that we whine and complain. It simply means we're humble to our bodies, we respect our feet, we respect the pain, and we respect our brilliant feedback mechanisms.

If something hurts, we stop. We analyze and change things accordingly. By being babies, we free ourselves from feeling the need to push through pain. We're not about running till we blister or break. Barefoot running's about being young again and experiencing the pure joy of the run.

It means when our feet, legs, or body are telling us something, we take note and listen carefully. It means we don't push into the danger zone, wondering if we'll feel better on the other side.

Instead we stop, go easy, or wait. By being humble, we keep our feet strong, our minds fresh, and our bodies happy.

Be Patient and Listen to Your Body

When it comes to transitioning into barefoot running, the tortoise will *always* beat the hare. So what's the easiest, safest, most effective way to transition? Take off the shoes cold turkey. No transition shoes, no easing in. Dive off the deep end and into the water.

But wait! You say. *Won't I get an overuse injury right away?*

Yes, if you don't listen to your body and go too far or too fast.

You have the most amazing biofeedback mechanism already built into you. It's your skin. Run too far on bare skin and blisters, and shredded feet, pureed skin, or tenderized pads coupled with thousands of nerve endings embedded in your feet will stop you in your tracks.

If you run too far barefoot one day, you'll certainly be unable to do it the next. But if you watch your feet, particularly your skin, you'll stop well in advance of pain.

As soon as your skin feels too sore, or you even whiff the hint of the first blister coming on, you should stop, put on your shoes (carry them with you initially as "hand weights"), and turn for home.

Let your skin be your guide. This skin advice goes beyond your first few excursions too. Let it be your guide for training in general. If your skin feels strong, head out on a run. If not, stay home.

Letting go of the outcome

When it comes to barefoot running, you need to let go of the outcome, which means letting go of goals, whether that's a time, fitness level, or future race. Transitioning into barefoot running is highly individual, though it usually takes 3 to 6 months, after which you'll be faster and stronger than ever before. Barefoot running is more than a sport; it's a dance with nature and the Universe to discover the capabilities of your body. It's a dance of being aware and letting go, turning things over to a higher power, or just to that still, small voice inside you.

I'm talking about going with the flow, or letting the Universe be your guide. This means *stop trying to drive the ship*. You'll find yourself in trouble when you command the ship and push too far, or too fast, or when you ignore that intuitive voice in your head. It's also why you need to be careful in competition, whether you're running against yourself, or against a watch, a deadline, a goal, or a race. It's in competition that you are most susceptible to letting your ego overshadow your instincts. You may drive yourself into the ground.

We're in school on this planet, learning to use time, space, and this temporary shell that I refer to as the "meat-suit." I'd love to know what we're capable of as humans, for I don't believe in limits. The only limits we have are those our minds set.

When we are barefoot running in solitude, it's a lot easier to stay in the "zone," in that quiet place where the material world fades away. Ego takes us out of the zone. It unplugs us from that silent inner voice and vetoes our awareness. We're no longer thinking about our breath, the road, glass, or our stride. Instead, we're intent on going longer, faster, and farther. And that's precisely when we run into trouble.

Letting go of expectation

Barefoot running is not about forcing things, but about flowing like water and letting nature guide you where she may. Some people, like Jessica, pick up barefoot running fast. Others, like myself, a bit more slowly. Some days you'll want to run long and fast. Other days you'll want to keep your runs short and sweet. When it comes to barefoot running, listen to the earth, to the stillness, to your body, and to the silence. Let these forces guide you along. If you go out without a plan, without any expectation, deadline, or specific goal in mind, it's amazing how far you'll travel and how fresh you'll be.

This is also the premise behind a beautiful book by Dr. Majid Ali called *The Ghoraa and Limbic Exercise*. He talks about how the African messenger lets go and can run effortlessly almost without breaking a sweat, mile after mile, while the American businessman labors, toils, and struggles to run at his doctor-prescribed 20 minutes at 70 percent of his maximal heart rate. The messenger lets go and can fly while the businessman, stuck focused on his goal, struggles and may even hurt himself.

Jessica learned this lesson of letting go as she started barefoot running. Sometimes she did a workout; other times she skipped or modified. Sometimes she went for a run, and on more than one occasion, a workout turned into a hike. It seemed disorganized and she called it "lazy" in the beginning. But letting go of the specifics and just doing what felt right helped her tremendously. Within 3 short months she could run up to 5 miles barefoot, and even ran the steepest trails along slickrock in Utah. All because she let nature guide her and went without a plan.

Having no expectation or plans is a plan unto itself—one of letting go. Without expectation we never push ourselves too far or too fast. We become one with the earth and simply flow.

So run without ego. Leave behind the desire to go "X" miles in "Y" minutes. There's nothing wrong with a training plan, but if you need to drop it, be courageous enough to do so. If you head out for 30 minutes but realize 5 minutes is all your feet can handle, take a break. If you're running with a group and the pace is too high, don't be afraid of dropping back. Conversely, if you're flying along and don't even feel the ground, don't be afraid to go a bit farther. Chances are that over time you'll far surpass the speed and distance you once thought possible for yourself.

PART II

Tear Off Your Shoes and Truly Feel the Earth Beneath Your Feet

Heaven is under our feet as well as over our heads.
—Henry David Thoreau

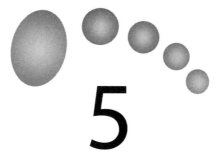

5

On Your Mark, Get Set, Get Those Shoes Off!

There's nothing like putting your bare feet into fresh cow dung on a cold day. It's great.

—Makhaya Ntini, South African athlete

Are you ready to wake up muscles and grow muscles that have been sleeping for years? It's time to retrain your body to move in ways it likely hasn't since you were a child. In the process, you'll gain better circulation. You'll strengthen all of your connective tissue and grow strong skin and protective padding on the bottoms of your feet.

But first, take the process slower than you ever imagined you were capable of going. Why? Because unlike muscles, which will feel relatively minimal strain in the upcoming training program, your ligaments and tendons have much more catching up to do and won't send as many warning signals. That's why runners often get into trouble. What we do today doesn't affect us for perhaps a week or two down the road. Fair warning!

This chapter is divided into two sections. In the first half, you can train yourself to become more aware of your mind and your body. By emptying your mind of thoughts, you free up space to listen to the many cues your body is constantly giving you. And by listening more carefully to your body, you enable yourself to provide a self-diagnosis and dictate the best custom-designed training program for yourself.

In the second half of this chapter, you will learn proper running form, keeping in mind there are two important areas to concentrate on. One, you will be encouraged to develop a natural alignment that minimizes overuse injuries. Two, you will be coached for the lightest, most efficient stride in order to minimize impact on your body.

Let's start with a preliminary self-assessment of your body!

Checking In: How Do You Feel?

Running barefoot is running aware. Do you know how your body feels right now? How are your feet, legs, lower back, and shoulders? Are you holding tension anywhere? Is anything sore or not quite right? You can't become the best runner of your life if you don't know your body. But don't worry, barefoot running and some simple exercises will help you reawaken self-awareness and your mind-body connection.

When you wake up in the morning, first step out of bed, or do a morning meditation, do you ever ask yourself, *How do I feel?* or *How am I doing?* Chances are, your body knows a lot more than you realize and it doesn't take rocket science to discover what it knows. The clues are always there, or as I like to say, *the answers are always on the inside.*

If we only listened to our bodies, we'd have a much better idea of how we're doing and what we should plan for the day. It's very simple. If you feel a tweak or the slightest twinge of pain, don't think about it or intellectualize. Just stop what you're doing. If you feel a bit worn down, this means you should take it easy.

Ultra-endurance athletes, who often run 100 miles at a time or spend days traversing the Sahara, may be the best at this. It's rare to find an ultra-runner who follows a strict, regimented training program. Instead, they religiously listen to their bodies and adjust their training accordingly.

Vetoing the body when running over 100, or even 200 miles per week, would come at a very hefty price. So ultra-endurance athletes don't rely on a daily schedule, with repeats or intervals one day, track the next, endurance the next, and so forth. Instead, they wake up, perhaps walk around or meditate, and ask themselves, *How do I feel? What does the body feel like doing today?*

One great example is Sammy Wanjiru, winner of the 2008 Olympic Marathon. He was born in Kenya but trains in Japan using their highly structured training programs. However, Sammy is known for taking days off if his body feels the need. Just prior to the Olympics, he skipped a day to rest when it rained. Sammy knows that you have to listen to your body and give it a break when it asks for one. Though he's very young by marathon standards (22 years of age), he knows the key to success isn't just hard work, but recovery, going slow, and listening to the body.

Exercise: Taking Inventory

Try this: The next time you wake up in the morning, lie in bed for a few extra minutes. Practice taking long slow deep diaphragmatic breaths. If you think you may fall back asleep in bed, then get up for a few minutes, lie on a yoga mat, and do this on the floor.

While you're breathing, try to empty your mind. Let go of all thoughts. If you hear a thought, notice it, or label it as "thought" as they do in many Buddhist meditation practices, then let it go. If this doesn't work, simply count between your breaths. For instance, inhale, 1, 2, 3. Exhale, 1, 2, 3.

After a few minutes, when the mind is clear, take inventory of yourself. Begin with your feet and work up through the body, examining each area in your mind between breaths.

As a barefoot runner you have great advantages as well as challenges compared to the shod runner. Advantage—you can feel the ground and your body more and adapt on the fly. Disadvantage—there is no protection if you're out when you should be home resting.

Exercise: Preflight Inspection

As a barefoot runner, it's essential to take stock. Start with your feet.

Try this: Take a deep breath, sense your feet, curl your toes if it helps, hold your breath, then exhale and relax. Repeat this several times and get in touch with your feet. How do they feel? Are the toes doing all right? How about all 28 bones in your feet and countless ligaments and tendons? How does the skin feel? Rotate your ankles too. Does everything move freely, or do you feel resistance or tension anywhere?

Next move upward through your legs. Take a deep breath and inspect your calves. Breathe in, contract your calves, then exhale. How do they feel? Next your shins, then knees, quads, hamstrings, glutes, and then move up and out of the legs. Continue moving up your lower back, chest, shoulders, arms, neck and everywhere, even your face, sinuses, and head.

Are you getting a good sense or feel of everything?

Next, ask yourself how energetic do you feel. Refreshed and relaxed? Did you get a good night's rest? Do you feel well fueled? Well hydrated?

Take mental notes. With practice, you'll start to know your body very well.

> It's like a pilot inspecting a plane before each and every flight. Soon with a quick check in the morning you'll know if your body is ready for a long flight, a quick dash, or a day of maintenance.

Be flexible. If your body wants the day off, be kind to yourself and give in! Never think of yourself as missing a workout, being "lazy," or going too easy. Instead look at these days as blessings in disguise. For these "gifts" help us grow stronger and faster, keep us from injury, and let us get other things done, too.

Personally, I check on my condition numerous times during the day. First, immediately upon waking. Next, right *before* my run. Then, *during* my run. I don't want to tune out my body as I see so many people doing at gyms with blaring headphones and TVs. Instead, I want to keep in touch and know how everything feels. To stay in the now, focus on your breath or your footfalls, and empty your mind. Then, when a thought comes to you, such as, *I think it's hurting just behind that toe*, you can take stock of the situation quickly. Did your form get lazy? Do you need to bring up your arms? Or maybe your new minimalist shoes just aren't working for you.

Listen to your body in each and every moment. Don't be afraid to skip a workout, change a workout, or even turn for home. You're not being lazy, but being smart. I've headed out anticipating tremendous workouts, only to turn around within the first half mile or less.

Of course, if I'm feeling good, I let myself go long as well. I just need to listen to the still voice inside. It's the one in touch with my body and with the Universe.

In the Zone

In Tibet, there once lived yogi runners called the Lung-Gom-Pa. These breath runners or trance runners (as they appeared to run in a trance) would travel incredible distances nearly barefoot, often with only straw sandals on their feet, and were reported to travel farther and faster than horses.

In the book *Tibetan Magic and Mysticism* by J.H. Brennan, there's a story of a group of people coming across a Lung-Gom-Pa runner, moving off in the distance, nearly as fast as their car. One passenger wanted to ask the runner questions, but another passenger quickly advised against it, explaining that the runner was running in a deep trance and that if he were disturbed, the God within him would depart and he might die.

Now, this warning could be taken as literal. Perhaps the runner was in such a meditative state—so at one with the Universe—that a break in concentration could send his spirit fleeing from his body. Or perhaps, more likely, a break in concentration at such high speed would send him careening out of control, tripping over rocks, and falling flat on his face.

I can only imagine what years of breath training and meditation might do for our ability to run far and run fast. For when we run at our best, we, too, are in a near meditative state. We're keenly aware of our surroundings, our breath, and our footfalls, but not of our thoughts, or our worries, or of showing off. We're simply one with the run and one with our breath. We're not running, but being the run, or as I've heard it described by yogis, Native Americans, and Mick Dodge, a natural movement expert in the Northwest, we're being pulled along by the power of the earth itself.

Mindful barefoot running and focusing on the breath puts us in the zone. When I'm in the zone, I feel the ground, yet don't. I'm acutely aware of everything beneath and around me, and of nothing at all. It feels as if I'm flying, hovering 2 feet above the ground in a trance, or a dreamlike state. At these times I've passed cyclists going uphill and I've felt I could catch my shadow running downhill. It's 100 percent speed, yet with zero percent effort. I feel as if I've "plugged in" and my body or feet are drawing immense energy from the ground.

Exercise: Warming Up

As in any sport or physical endeavor, warming up is essential if you plan on staying injury-free. You can start with a few light drills, barefoot walking, or a few foot-muscle strengthening exercises. The more warmed up and relaxed your muscles are, the more likely you'll find yourself in near perfect barefoot running form.

Whether you're an experienced veteran barefoot runner, or a newbie just getting into the game, I recommend warming up slowly. Check out professional runners and you'll see them walking along for 5 or 10 minutes before they hit their stride.

Personally, I like to walk into my runs, slowly moving along, gaining a head of steam, and then, when the going feels right, break into a light jog. Sometimes it's just a few minutes, sometimes quite a bit more.

If it's really cold out, I'll even start walking, and then jogging, in shoes. Once my feet are loose and warm, but before they start sweating, I strip off the shoes, and I'm ready to go.

◐°°°₀ FOOT NOTE: Head Uphill

Want the simplest, easiest way to warm up? Walk up a hill. It's a natural way to warm up, and you'll soon find yourself breaking into a sweat and then jog, all with minimal effort.

Walking uphill to warm up puts minimal stress on your joints and is a workout unto itself. If you're just getting started, there's nothing wrong with walking up the hill, and if it's long enough (one-half mile or longer), just walk home and call it good.

Grass for Starters

Although I like beginners to feel a hard surface, a swath of 50 to 100 yards of gently sloped park or well-groomed grassy area is sufficient for your first few efforts. You can even begin on AstroTurf or a well-groomed baseball field. A soft surface is fine, as long as it's smooth. If it's uneven or rough terrain, it's not going to help you begin.

Why not run straight on a hard path? I don't think there's anything wrong with it. But there's something incredibly fun and special about starting on the grass. It makes us all feel like kids again and feels great beneath our feet. So I start all of my clinics on grass; then after some drills, we progress out onto sidewalks and bike paths.

Hard surfaces are ideal for building technique quickly. They force you to feel the ground and find the lightest, softest step possible. But I like starting runners briefly on soft surfaces in the beginning, it's just more fun. And that's what barefoot running is all about—focusing on the fun.

The grass may be softer, but it's not actually easier on the muscles. Instead, the uneven ground beneath grass helps you gain some muscle strength before forcing them to do something that really taxes the muscles a lot. Over time, running on grass becomes a great uneven surface for working on muscle strength, core strength, and form.

Exercise: Get Scrunching

Let's warm up your feet with a fun little exercise. This is one of our favorite activities at our clinics. It warms up the feet, strengthens the arches, and gets you ready for your barefoot runs.

Try this: Get a golf ball and start working on picking it up with your toes. Practice this before each of your runs to warm up your feet. You can try this every day to strengthen your arches. Work on grabbing the ball with your toes. Notice how your arch naturally raises and tightens? Just as you lift weights to tone arms, legs, or even abs, you can build those arches by grabbing with your toes.

If you're recovering from injury or plantar fasciitis, just be wise. Never go to

---

the point of pain, and if there's a dull ache, STOP. You're probably not ready.

For your first time, start with a minute at most of scrunching the ball, and that's it. Then rest before trying this exercise again. The next time you pick up the golf ball, try it for 2 minutes, then rest, then perhaps 3, and so forth. Before you know it, you'll almost be juggling with your feet and your happy, healthy arches.

Mindful Running

Thich Nhat Hanh, a Vietnamese Buddhist monk and author of *The Miracle of Mindfulness*, teaches that being mindful means being in the moment, being aware, and being at one with whatever it is you're doing, even if it's washing the dishes.

I'm often found in a state of mindfulness while running, similar to the Lung-Gom-Pa runners from Tibet and the Marathon Monks of Mount Hiei in Japan. It's said that as they traverse the same marathon loop daily, the Marathon Monks are so present and aware of their surroundings, they know every rock and twig on their path. They know when each bird wakes in the morning. And just by watching the clouds, they can forecast the weather a week in advance.

When I run barefoot, I empty my mind and focus on being one with my environment. To do this, I use the following 3 basic techniques: focusing on the breath, focusing on a distant object, and remaining in a state of thanks.

Focusing on the breath

I look at the mind as a muscle and thinking as weightlifting. If you were to lift weights continuously 16 hours per day, your muscles would cramp up and cease to function. It's the same with thought. If we don't give our brains a chance to rest and relax, they seize and turn to mush. We need quality over quantity in our training, both of body and mind. Giving the brain a chance to relax on our runs adds to the quality of our thought, work, and all interactions throughout the day.

And that's without considering the fantastic benefits we get from the endorphins released in our brains when we run. Endorphins are proteins that give us focus, relax our minds, and reduce tension and pain throughout our day. They don't call it a "runner's high" for nothing. It's likely that the release of endorphins originally evolved to help us run and hunt longer to bring food home for the tribe.

Exercise: Running Without Thought

Try this: While feeling the ground with your feet, focus on each inhalation and exhalation. With each exhalation let more of your mind chatter go. If you catch yourself thinking about anything, simply label the thoughts as "thinking," and without any judgments, let the thought(s) go and return to your breath.

This is difficult to do at first, but over time you'll start catching your thoughts sooner and sooner, until it comes very quickly. This is another practice found in many Buddhist traditions, but you don't need to be a Buddhist to practice it.

You can do this whenever you're running, whether on a city street, in a park, or out in nature. It helps you empty the mind and simply be one with the trail, the earth, and the run. In our crazy, hectic lives, having even 30 minutes of down time to let go of thought and relax the mind can be an amazing gift. Couple that with a fantastic barefoot run, and you may find nirvana just outside your door.

Focusing on a distant object

Lung-Gom-Pa runners use a similar technique to this exercise by focusing on a distant star as they run in the night. Then even if the star sets and they're still running, they imagine the star in front of them, just below the horizon. Focusing on a star keeps you light and helps you float, almost above the ground. It's been said if you clear your mind and focus on a star, it will almost carry you along and give you energy.

Exercise: Grounding in the Moment

Try this: Focus on a star in front of you. Picture this star while letting go of all other thought. Simply focus all your attention on this star. I like repeating a mantra in my head in time with each breath, such as, "Thank you for this beautiful star." Focusing on an object before you keeps your mind from wandering and grounds you in the moment.

Remaining in a state of thanks

I use this third meditation technique throughout my day. Despite my diagnosis of ADHD (attention deficit hyperactivity disorder), to help me stay focused and in the moment, I made some beaded bracelets, which I call my Barefoot Beads. By running my fingers along each individual bead, it helps me remain in a quiet, aware, yet meditative state.

I typically repeat the following mantra-like statements, over and over, throughout my runs or throughout my day:

Thank you for this beautiful day. Thank you for this beautiful day. Thank you for this beautiful day. Or Thank you for this beautiful run. Thank you for this beautiful run. Thank you for this beautiful run.

Staying in the moment is particularly important in barefoot running where one stumble or misplaced step could hurt badly. Yet when I'm mindful and focused, I'm more aware of my surroundings, the environment, the terrain, and my two feet.

Exercise: Express Gratitude While Running

Try this: While placing your attention on the tree (or rock or other marker) 50 to 100 feet in front of you, repeat a mantra such as, "Thank you for this beautiful tree." Being in a state of gratitude, whether giving thanks for the tree, the life force all around you, the earth you're running on, or this beautiful day, helps block out extraneous thoughts and keeps you in the moment.

When I'm feeling the earth while running barefoot in nature, I'm in awe and thankful for everything, but especially to be alive.

Step-by-Step Guide to Proper Barefoot Running Form

Barefoot running starts with your head—what's inside your head—as you are preparing to begin. Now you can also prepare to run lighter than ever before. We will start at the waist and move up.

Yes, eventually, we will get to the all-important foot strike, stride, and mechanics of the foot itself. But running erect is equally as important as running with proper stride and foot strike. When you stand tall in a proper position, you help the rest of your stride fall naturally into place. These are the 5 key elements of proper upper-body positioning:

1. Keeping your **pelvis** in neutral alignment

2. Engaging your **core**

3. Opening your **chest**

4. Standing with a tall **spine**

5. Positioning your **arms**

Keeping it neutral—your pelvic tilt

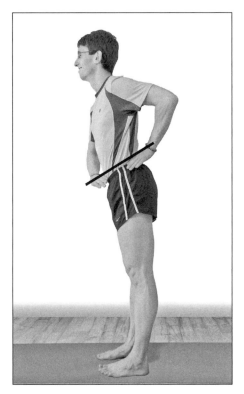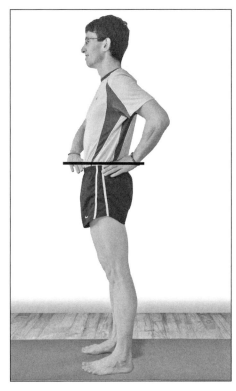

Avoid an awkward forward bend—a common habit developed through modern running shoes. To break this habit, work to get your pelvis neutral by placing one hand in front and one behind you at waist height. With each hand in position, work to bring them level or even in height. This is your strongest running position and least likely to get you injured.

You've seen them running everywhere—people with their butts sticking out. You can't run well if you're sticking out your butt. I've seen several of my students lean forward from their upper body, yet remain vertical below the waist. In essence, they're collapsing their upper bodies forward while pivoting at the hip. This creates the butt problem.

Make sure your waist is level and your pelvis is not dipping forward. Unfortunately, high heels, dress shoes, and especially today's taller running shoes have habitualized a slightly forward dipping pelvic tilt.

If you run with this tilt, you can't use your core as an anchor and you can't take advantage of gravity. Instead by bending at the waist, you wreak havoc on your center of gravity. You have made yourself an inefficient runner, and over time you risk causing great damage.

By leaning forward at the waist, you place undue force on your quadriceps, knees, shins, and ankles, changing the force dynamics through the foot, and dangerously overstretching and straining your hamstrings. This explains why you see so many runners with hamstring injuries.

To correct this problem you must become conscious of your pelvic tilt. Try the following exercise.

Exercise: Imagery

Try this: Picture your pelvis as a giant bowl filled to the rim with water. Lean too far forward and the imaginary water swooshes forward out of the bowl. Lean too far backward and the water swooshes out in the opposite direction. Instead, you want the bowl (or pelvis) nice and neutral with the front of your waist the same height as the back of your waist. This imagery helps you stand perfectly erect.

Place one hand in front of your waist and one hand behind, both hands just above the hips. Check to see if your hands are level with each other. Is the front lower than the back? Then tilt your pelvis back. Is the back hand lower than the front? Then tilt your pelvis forward.

If you're still struggling with this one, you're not alone. It often helps to practice this exercise while standing in front of a mirror with your shirt off. Pilates classes can also help you learn how to get in a pelvis neutral position. Also, you can try standing on a small inflatable balance cushion. This is my favorite for working on pelvic positioning while strengthening the core.

Snap your belly button to your spine

Your core (abdominals and back muscles) is where you develop your true power, balance, and grace. Running barefoot is all about using gravity and running from your core, rather than from your legs. Your core, or the combination of your belly and your back, acts as your anchor. Running from the core helps keep you tall, stable, and injury-free. In essence, your core is your foundation.

When you're shod, your footwear also attempts to hold you upright and balanced in position, albeit quite precariously. Without footwear, our own bodies and skeletons are responsible for keeping us upright, stable, and in proper alignment. This is important for balance and for letting gravity do the work. Your core now takes on the bulk of this responsibility, as it should, which is why you need to spend more time strengthening your core.

Ideally, you're aiming to build all movement and activity upon a strong core. To aid in this process, I highly recommend practicing balance exercises which I'll discuss later. Also, consider signing up for a Pilates class. (I prefer Pilates exercises over countless sit-ups and crunches, as these allow you to cheat and don't properly engage your muscles in ways we can use them while barefoot running.) For now, use this imagery exercise to engage your core.

Exercise: Snap Your Belly Button

Try this: Picture an imaginary giant metal clothing snap, about 6 inches in diameter. The front of the snap is centered on your belly button. The back of the snap is centered on the small of your back at your spine. Now, snap the two pieces together or snap your belly button to your spine; you'll pull in your gut, pull in your back, and snap them both together.

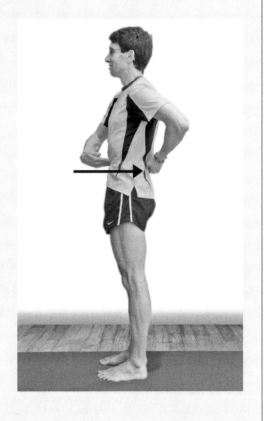

This exercise will help you bring in both your belly and your back, producing a nice, very gentle arch in your back. If you were to lie down with your belly button snapped to your spine, you'd actually find a pocket or small arch in the back through which you could slide your hand. This action holds everything tight to keep the body from moving from side to side, as you swing your arms and legs in opposition as balanced pendulums swinging from a strong base.

As you tighten your core, it's important to remember to stay relaxed and continue breathing. Be careful not to hold your breath. Instead, keep your chest rising and falling naturally, while focusing on pulling in the muscles beneath the chest and lungs.

Grasp the idea of snapping your belly button to your spine, and you've just saved yourself from a plethora of potential injuries and future doctors' bills.

Open your chest

Humans are the only true bipeds. Standing or moving upright on two legs gives us the ability to breathe without restriction as our arms and legs move. Our ability to adjust our breathing patterns according to speed, terrain, heat, and stress is unique in the animal kingdom. This is one reason you hear about humans outrunning horses over great distances, or why indigenous peoples are able to run down animals in persistence hunting. Let's make the best of our biological advantage and open up our chests and lungs.

Exercise: Inflate the Balloon

Try this: Keep your belly in, while bringing your chest up and wide. Picture your chest filled with two balloons, one on each side, or one giant balloon, expanding and contracting with each breath. The bigger you practice inflating the balloons, the more air you'll take in for each and every stride.

Your chest adapts over time, growing stronger and wider for each breath. As you learn to coordinate a tightened core with expanded lungs (belly in, lungs expanded), you become an incredible breath machine, drawing fantastic power from the air, while remaining firmly anchored and perfectly erect.

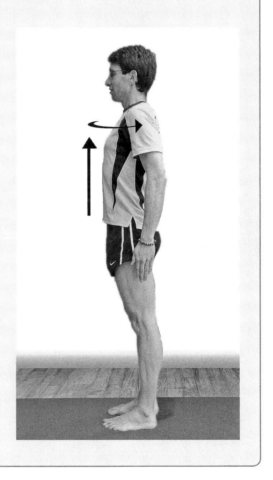

Here's one thing to watch for. When you "open up" your chest by bringing it up and wide, you may feel inclined to raise or shrug your shoulders. This action tenses and strains the shoulders, back, and neck, while throwing you off balance. Don't hunch your shoulders in an effort to counter this. Instead, keep them down and relaxed. Shrugged or hunched shoulders constrict your breathing and throw off your arm movement resulting in a choppy, unnatural, imbalanced stride. Breathe easy by keeping those shoulders relaxed.

Silvery string to the sky

Now that your body is in proper alignment, you will want to pull yourself up nice and tall so you're incredibly light on your feet.

Exercise: Silver String

Try this: Picture an imaginary silver string. The string starts at your feet, passes through your tailbone, spine, chest, neck, and through the center of your head. This string will keep you light on your toes and help you maintain proper position and balance.

With an imaginary fishing reel, wind that string tight, and pull yourself tall as if you're being yanked up so high you're almost pulled onto your tiptoes.

Keep your head facing forward and your jaw relaxed. Remember, the string pulls up through the center of your head, not the front.

You'll always want to run with this silvery string pulling you to the sky.

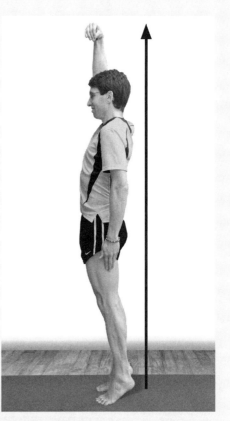

Our bodies also have memories—meaning what we do when we're not running carries through to our stride. From now on you'll always want to stand, and even sit, as tall as possible (with your core engaged). Try to stand this tall in all activities throughout your day.

Before you begin running, always pull yourself up as tall as you can. You can even pull yourself up onto the very tips of your toes, before lowering your feet back down and preparing to begin.

Bring your arms up into a W

The arms are very important for all running, and in particular for barefoot running. Why? Because your arms drive your legs. Your arms and legs move in near-perfect opposition as well-balanced counterweights. Whatever your right arm does, your left leg does, and vice versa. And when you're barefoot, you will feel the consequences of subtle changes even more. A slightly dropped right arm means you feel the effects significantly in the stride of the left leg.

To set the stage for a proper stride, in this exercise, bring your arms up to help them "fall" into a more symmetrical, natural position by your sides. Then you're only a few steps away from your lightest run ever!

Exercise: Think WoW

Try this: Bring your arms up above your head and out to the side in the shape of a W. This allows you to naturally bend your arms at a 90-degree angle without rolling your shoulders in or pinning them back. Next, drop your arms to your sides. Your arms are now naturally in a good starting position.

Avoid shrugging or raising your shoulders in an effort to bring your arms into proper position. The shoulders should remain nice and relaxed with all movement swinging off the shoulders, not *from* shoulder movement.

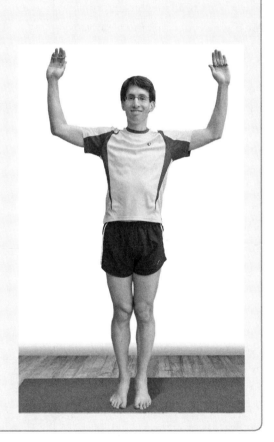

Let's review: Snap your belly in. Then pull your chest up. Next, widen your shoulders, or as they say in Pilates and my instructor Don Spence used to say, bring yourself in, up, and wide.

- In—Snap the belly button to your back.

- Up—Bring your chest up as high as you can.

• Wide—Widen your shoulders as if they're the wings on a plane.

Keeping your core in the strongest position possible helps open up the breathing passages for air. So focus on being in, up, and wide at all times.

Spring-load your chicken wings

Once you're in, up, and wide with that string pulling to the sky, and you've made your giant W, you want to spring-load your arms at 90-degree angles to form spring-loaded chicken wings.

I call the arms spring-loaded chicken wings for a couple of reasons. First, you're going to look like an overstuffed chicken running with your arms in this position, but that's okay because it's the most efficient position. Second, by keeping your arms pulled back, with the tiniest bit of tension in your back, you bring your chest forward, keeping you light and springy on your feet.

Running barefoot requires you to keep your legs up high, which helps you stay light on your feet. To do this, keep your arms up high and at a 90-degree bend, if not greater. The higher you keep your arms, the higher you keep your legs. I even encourage runners to over-exaggerate their arms by keeping them above 90 degrees. This is done to compensate for what naturally occurs when you increase your speed, which is to drop your arms a bit.

To begin, we're aiming for perfect symmetry—and high arms.

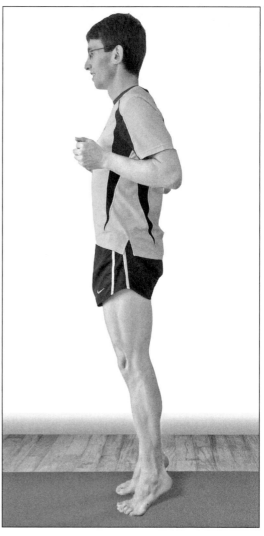

Chicken wings: Drop your arms down from their W, keeping a 90-degree bend or greater. While standing tall, bring your arms back slightly to create your spring-loaded chicken wings.

Exercise: Spring-load Your Chicken Wings

Try this: Picture two loops sewn into the armpits of your shirt, one on each side. With your hands as loosely clenched fists, bring your forearms up to form a 90-degree angle. Now hook your thumbs into each of these loops. You want your hands to be just in front of your chest, an inch or so above your nipple line, or as close to the height of your armpits as you can get them. Your elbow should be pulled close to your sides, but without any great tension on your shoulders or back to hold them close. Your arms should be pulled back, with just a bit of tension.

To start your arm swing, rotate your arm and fist toward your ears, then down toward your back. You want to use the minimum movement necessary to help propel you forward so don't exaggerate the swing or over-rotate.

Make sure your arms never travel below a perpendicular line to the ground. Always keep your elbows bent at 90 degrees or less with your gently closed hands or fists up by your armpits and never drop them toward the ground. Then swing gently, like a pendulum. Let your arms move naturally forward and back in rhythm with your opposing leg. Keep them up high to keep your legs up high. Always track them forward and backward, never to the sides, as you want to drive all of your energy forward, rather than wasting energy in side-to-side movement.

Bringing your arms across your body, rather than forward, is a very common mistake resulting in lost efficiency and potentially injury. Crossing arms forces your core to work overtime to keep you from swaying. This crossover is potentially dangerous because wherever your arm goes, your leg is sure to follow. Crossed arms pull your legs in and can rotate your feet, straining your feet and arches and putting undue stress and rotational force on your hips, IT bands, knees, and more.

On this note, make sure you're swinging from relaxed shoulders and not from the back. There should be no rotational or side-to-side movement of the shoulders or the back. Check that your shoulders stay wide but relaxed and without excess motion. Rotating your shoulders to the side puts significant, potentially damaging rotational force on your back and neck. Swinging your arms does not mean swinging your shoulders.

Note: Surely you see runners with an iPod or water bottle in just one hand. They're at great risk of an overuse injury because they're dropping one arm and slightly twisting their body to the side. This doesn't just affect their back, shoulders, and neck, but the twisting continues through the hips, and asymmetry continues right down through their legs.

Running barefoot helps you become aware of imbalances and asymmetries, but since your arms drive your legs, you need to watch your arms. Therefore, if you carry something in the right hand, I highly recommend you have a matching weight or object in your left hand. Even the weight of a watch worn on one wrist can make a difference, particularly the older, heavier GPS's and altimeters. Think symmetry.

Less is more: Moving your arms at speed

Sprinters drive their arms forward toward the finish line. As you run faster, your arms naturally swing farther and farther. However, with a barefoot runner's fast cadence, your arms needn't move as far as a shod runner's arms. Instead, a barefoot runner's arms will always be closer and tighter to the body. This reduces excess movement, again making you more efficient than your shod counterparts. Experiment with your swing as you increase speed to find a balance between driving yourself forward and conserving energy. Keep the arms up and think minimal movement. Period.

> ## *Exercise:* Towel Run
>
> **Try this:** If you're struggling to keep your arms up high, try running with a short towel draped around your neck. Hold the towel with each hand so your arms can't move more than an inch or two in front of you. Work on keeping your arms up nice and high without any side-to-side movement. Soon enough, you'll be running without the towel and keeping your arms up high.

○°°˳ FOOT NOTE

On downhills: Never drop your arms on a downhill. Wherever your arms go, your body is sure to follow; if you drop your arms, your body droops forward, putting more pressure, rather than less, on your knees and joints. Instead keep the arms high, stay tall and erect, and let a gentle lean back slow you down. Never forget the silvery string pulling you tall on downhills.

Put Your Best Stride Forward

Barefoot running is about getting your feet out in front of you and landing light on your forefoot. Let's practice landing on your toes.

Barefoot running requires taking short, quick strides. Think of taking small pitter-patter spring-loaded steps with your feet out a foot in front of you. You'll find that the spring comes naturally, as landing on your forefoot gives you the sensation of bouncing along off your toes, feet, and calves. However, you don't want to bounce high or over-exaggerate this. Over time, you'll want your head to remain level, with no excess movement.

Exercise: Jog Light

Try this: With your body in proper alignment, gently jog down your gentle park slope (perhaps only a 1 percent incline though flat will do too), springing off each foot, staying nice and light, and going slow. Keep thinking "light" to yourself, moving forward with as little effort or bounce as possible. You should continue for 50 to 100 yards or about the length of a football field—and then stop. Turn around and "Tiger Walk" (explained next) back to your starting point.

Because 18 of 19 tendons of your feet are connected to your toes, working your toes strengthens almost every muscle of the foot. Use the Tiger Walk imagery to help you run stronger and build better arches and gain proper form for when your feet hit the ground. This advanced, moving version of the golf-ball scrunch helps dynamically build your arch while training it to be strong when you hit the ground. Every beginner practices this exercise during our clinics.

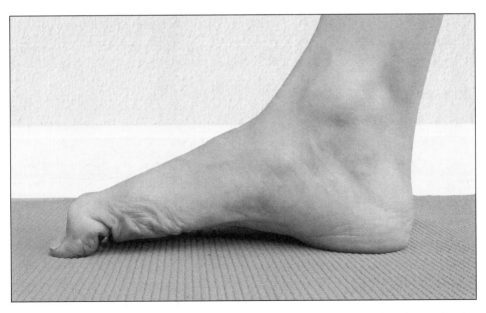

Walk like a tiger: Imagine you have tiger paws and tiger claws. With each step, land lightly either flat or just slightly on your forefoot. Grab the ground with your claws and dig in—a movement designed to pull up (and thereby strengthen) your arch.

Exercise: Tiger Walk

Try this: Pretend you're a tiger walking with your claws extended, grabbing the ground, and pulling through with each stride. With your imaginary claws, grab with your toes into the ground. Spread your toes apart and, with each step, land on your forefoot with your heel slightly lifted off the ground and pull forward with your claws. I recommend integrating this exercise into your warm-up program, indoors or outdoors.

Now that you've jogged 50 to 100 yards and then tiger walked back, let's repeat. Turn around, pull yourself even taller, snap that belly button to the spine again, open up your chest, and widen your shoulders. Repeat your 50–100 yard jog, followed by the Tiger Walk.

For the first day, you should do no more than 5 or 6 efforts of both the Tiger Walk and the light jog, and that's it. Err on the short side, and if you start getting sore, stop. Enjoy the ear-to-ear grin you're likely sporting and head for home.

If you want, jog lightly for your last effort on a bike path or sidewalk next to the park to "feel the ground." Then go home, you're done.

You can even use the Tiger Walk for your walks home and even in your shoes, as long as there is ample room in the toe box to spread your toes. One good time to do the Tiger Walk is when you're fatigued from running. Turn around and head for home, then walking along, grab the ground with your tiger paws and claw yourself home. It'll give your feet one of the greatest workouts in the world!

Don't twist and shout

Running barefoot allows you to run efficiently, light, and without wasted energy. Often, runners waste energy moving side to side and up and down. Just watch runners going by the next time you're out on a path, street, or trail. Do they swing their hips or arms to the sides? Are they bouncing up and down? Or does their foot kick out or to the side at the end of their stride?

With barefoot running, the technique is to get all of your energy moving forward, *not* up and down, and *not* side to side. Feeling the ground makes it vastly easier for you to take note of your movements. Going barefoot helps you quiet your stride, become silky smooth, and erase excess movement. What's excess? Any movement that doesn't carry you forward. If you swing to the side, you must counterbalance that weight by pulling to the other side. If you bounce up and down, not only do you waste energy going up, you must also absorb extra force upon each landing. None of this effort carries you forward.

The average runner bounces up and down about 3 inches per stride. Over the course of a marathon, that little 3-inch bounce accumulates to more than a mile of vertical distance. No wonder a marathon's so exhausting! Running 26.2 miles is one thing, but simultaneously running up Pike's Peak? That's a lot of wasted energy. Just think how much faster and fresher you'd be if you simply cut that bounce in half.

The more you practice your form, the more you'll see proper, and not-so-proper, form in others. Paying closer attention to your body, and watching the form of others will help instruct and remind you of your own proper form. Become an artist of your sport and start studying other runners, both recreational and professional.

Watch to see what wasted movement looks like versus efficient striding. Then watch yourself running in a mirror such as on a treadmill, in a dance hall, or in front of shop windows. Better still, practice these 3 exercises: Shadow Stalker, Wall Bounce, and Long-Distance Stare.

Exercise: Shadow Stalker

Try this: Try to run directly behind your shadow just after sunrise or before the sun sets. Do you see any bounce up and down or sway to the sides? Does it look as if you have a dancing partner rather than a shadow? Or does your shadow appear to be riding a pogo stick? If so, engage your core, hold yourself in proper position, and see if the shadow's movement changes. Over time, work to minimize any shadow movement that's not directly heading forward.

Exercise: Wall Bounce

Try this: Run next to a wall or tall fence. Do you see the wall moving up and down beside you? Work to minimize the movement you see. The less movement of the wall, the less bounce in your stride.

Exercise: Long-Distance Stare

Try this: As you're running along, focus on an object just above the horizon at least 50 to 100 feet away, such as a distant street sign or a 10-foot-high tree branch. You'll notice that as you run, the sign bounces up and down, a reflection of your own bouncing.

Now work to stabilize the sign. The less the sign moves, the less your body moves. Practice this for a few minutes on every run. Better still, use this exercise as a meditation: focus on distant objects to help smooth your stride and quiet your mind.

Eliminate head wag

If your head is moving from side to side when you run, you've got head wag. We've all seen the "tail that wags the dog." In this case, wagging your head moves your entire body. As you run, work to keep your head tracking straight. This is exceptionally important, as your head is your anchor, like the tail of a dog.

Check out an online video of Haile Gebrselassie running. Notice his head movement or lack thereof. Haile doesn't bounce, wiggle, lean, or cock his head. His amazing neck muscles, which hold his head in place, are part of what gives him greatness, as he uses his head as an anchor for speed and stability. Work to eliminate head wag and make your head an anchor too.

Excess movement creates injuries and fatigue. When you're barefoot, it's easier to eliminate excess movement because you're more aware. Over time, you'll increase awareness of your feet and any bouncing, wiggling, head wagging, or arm dropping.

Let's go to the videotape

At our training camps and clinics, we often videotape our runners. Spotting inefficient movement on tape goes a long way toward helping runners correct their form. See if you can get a friend to videotape you as you run in the park or even on a treadmill. Then check out your stride and become familiar with it.

The more you watch yourself and others, the more you learn good form and catch your "mistakes." Personally, I tape myself at least once a month to improve my stride and eliminate excess motion. We can all benefit from a little glance in the mirror or a rewind of the tape.

Practicing good form isn't just for running. Muscle learning and memory takes place throughout your entire day. You can practice proper alignment at your desk in your chair, walking down the hall, or even in aisle 8 of your grocery store. The supermarket or shopping experience can be the perfect place to work on posture, core strength, and proper form.

Exercise: Toe Walking

Try this: The next time you're at a supermarket, picture that imaginary silvery string pulling up through your feet, your spine, your chest, shoulders, neck, and head up into the sky. It even pulls you right up onto the tips of your toes. Snap in your gut, pull yourself high, and walk around the supermarket an inch taller. Feel the difference? The more you do this, the better your overall posture and the better your running form.

Want an additional challenge? Don't mind the strange looks? Walk a bit on your toes, almost as if you're in heels, but with nothing beneath you (don't forget to grab and scrunch with your toes as you go along). This strengthens your calves, feet, and arches and gets you in the most natural position of them all. After all, it's how our kids begin walking before we put them in shoes.

Toe walking helps you stay tall, quiet, and in the best form for healthy walking and running. It's not just the best runners who make no sound, but the best walkers too.

Hand Weights aka Shoes

When I begin a clinic, I always pick up a pair of shoes and give a pop quiz. *What are these?* I ask, pointing to my shoes.

Torture devices? Maybe. *Cruelty chambers?* Certainly. *Ways to get injured.* You bet! But most of all, they're hand weights!

Consider minimalist shoes as not only safety devices but also as your new hand weights. For all runners, and in particular beginners, whether running challenging terrain, extreme temperatures, or almost any other conditions, I recommend carrying footwear with you when you run.

This serves 3 main purposes:

1. When the going gets tough or you've fatigued and need to turn around, or if you run into any unexpected obstacles or challenges, you can throw on the shoes and safely get home.

2. Shoes are great hand weights you can use to help balance yourself and hold yourself in position. Holding something in your hands gives you a better kinesthetic feel for your body and position. It's easy to see where your arms and hands are by the height of your shoes in front of you, and you'll note if you're moving your arms and hands efficiently.

3. Hand weights build strength and endurance throughout your upper body including your biceps, triceps, chest, back, and even shoulders.

Shoes are also great in the winter for warming up the feet. When the pavement or trail's well below freezing, I like to begin my run in a minimalist shoe. Once the feet warm up, I peel off the shoes and use them as hand weights. If the feet get too cold, or if there's deep snow or ice ahead, I can simply slip them back on.

So bring those hand weights with you—for all the right reasons.

Barefoot Beads

When I'm not carrying "hand weights," I'm carrying my Barefoot Beads. Carrying beads is a simple way to remain mindful and work on technique without any substantial effort. As I run, I repeat a mantra while moving the beads of my bracelets through my hands. It helps me keep my arms relaxed and stay in a meditative state.

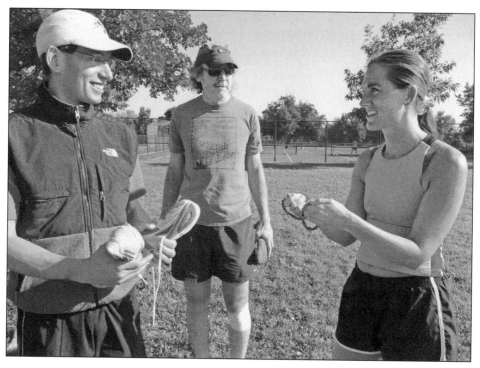

Barefoot running beads: Michael demonstrates the technique of using the barefoot running beads he developed. Hold the beads nice and light as you run with little bounce. Move the beads between your fingers as you repeat a mantra.

Carrying Barefoot Beads has an additional benefit over carrying hand weights. Holding beads lightly in your hands helps you see when you're bouncing. I'll often carry the beads loosely to see how little they can move in my hands. The less they move, the more efficiently I'm running. At the same time, holding beads loosely helps keep me from running with a clenched fist or dropping my hands, two big no-no's. Clenching your fists causes your entire body to tighten, and dropping the hands drops your entire body forward.

Michael's 2-Question Rule

Now that we've got you started, here's a very important rule I always teach my runners about when to go home. If you're tired and thinking of heading for home, feel sore, achy, or tender, or even have an inkling of doubt, ask yourself,

Should I stop? If the answer is yes, then head straight home, but chances are you'll say no and want to continue a little bit further.

At this point, double-check your form, go through the checklist for proper running form, and make sure you've re-snapped your belly button to your spine, re-sprung your chicken wings, and are staying tall. Did the soreness or fatigue go away? If so, great. If not, the next time you ask, *Should I stop?* Don't even finish the question, just turn around and head for home.

While the first question may be a fluke, the second time you ask if you should stop, it's your intuition that's connected to your body and your surroundings saying, *You've had enough, let's go home. Please* don't ignore it!

Don't be afraid to use this rule religiously. The 2-Question Rule will keep you out of harm's way!

Checklist for Proper Barefoot Running Form

Before you head out the door, review these key points.

☐ Scrunch It—Warm-up with Golf Ball Scrunches and Tiger Walking.

☐ Get Neutral—Neutralize your pelvic position by imagining your pelvis as a water bowl.

☐ Snap It In—Snap in your belly button to your spine.

☐ Open Up—Keep your chest up and open.

☐ Get Wide—Keep your shoulders wide and relaxed.

☐ Stand Tall—Imagine a silvery string pulling you tall.

☐ Raise Your Arms—Position your arms in a W above your head.

☐ Drop the Ws—Drop your arms to 90-degree angles by your side.

☐ Spring Load—Slightly pull back and spring-load your chicken wings for a slight forward lean.

☐ Don't Bounce—Be aware of excess movement by practicing Shadow Stalker and/or Long-Distance Stare.

☐ Stay Symmetrical—Consider bringing your hand weights (shoes) or Barefoot Beads to help keep things in check.

☐ Stay Relaxed and Have Fun—If you tense up, you're fighting against your body and the terrain. Keep your head, jaw, neck, shoulders, and every part of you relaxed. Instead of tensing, flow with the ground and with your form.

Congratulations! You're well on your way to exploring this fantastic new and eternally old way of running. It's as if you're peeking into Pandora's barefoot running box, and there's no turning back. You'll never view your form, nor anyone else's, in quite the same way. And you'll never run the same way again. Welcome to your new world, a world with a new form, new stride, and new possibilities.

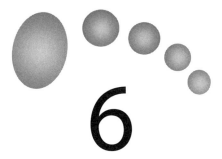

6

Anatomy of the Barefoot Strike and Stride

I think the secret of my light, quick, foot strike is related to the fact that I have fragile feet.

—Frank Shorter

When you're running barefoot, you're running on your forefoot, engaging a massive natural spring that begins with your forefoot and your arch and travels to your Achilles, calf, quad, glute, and even hamstring.

When you land on your forefoot, you engage all of this natural spring mechanism, but when you land on your heel or midfoot (with your heel down), you lock out your protective mechanism. Instead, you become 100 percent reliant on the cushioning of the shoe. (Even an inch of shoe cushioning pales in comparison to the 2- or 3-foot-long spring of your leg.)

The English expression "to stay on your toes" implies that you'd better stay alert. Staying on your toes allows you to make quick adjustments. It's why you see ballet dancers, gymnasts, and kung fu masters spending so much time on their toes. It's also why you see football players practicing lateral movement tire drills on their toes. They hop side to side and in and out of tires, all while balancing on their toes.

Perhaps, Dr. Marc Silberman, founder of the NJ Sports Medicine and Performance Center, puts it best, "You'd never see a 3-, 4-, or 5-year-old running across the street on their heels, nor would you jump rope, hop off a stool or a ladder, box, dribble a soccer ball, nor take a jump shot, nor would you ever run uphill while running on your heels.

So why would we strike our heels repetitively while running?"

Running on your toes not only prevents bone-jarring shock from traveling all the way up your spine, but also eliminates it in the first place. And it's springy too! Check out Haile Gebrselassie, world's fastest marathoner, or almost any great track runner these days. They're all on their toes.

Why? Because toe running is faster, lighter, and makes you more nimble. It's also more efficient and prevents shock. When you land on your toes, you land like a ballet dancer, with your foot out in front of you. Essentially, you're engaging in a controlled lunge. You absorb all impact with your muscles, not with your joints. And you don't just absorb the shock, you load it into the muscles to spring you back at the end of your stride.

Imagine no more air, gel, coils, or other inventions to absorb the shock pounding through your heels. Instead, you employ nature-made springs that effortlessly help you bound forward with every stride.

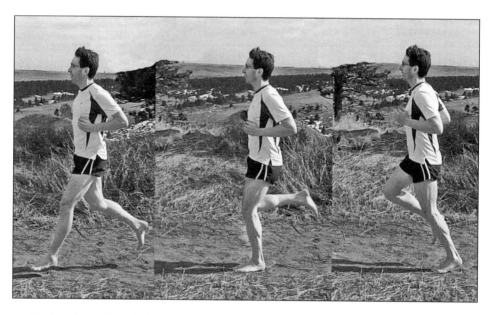

Ideal strike and stride length: (1) Extend your leg, preparing to grab with your toes. (2) Land lightly on your forefoot with the leg perpendicular to the ground. (3) Bring your opposing leg up and through quickly, thinking fast, light and easy strides.

(Observation: though I have contacted the ground with my forefoot first, it compresses down to absorb energy and rebound for a softer, smoother, more efficient stride. This comes over time with additional foot, Achilles, and calf strength.)

But wait, there's more, as they say on the TV infomercials! Here's another bonus, free with barefoot running: You add several inches to your inseam when you run on your toes. This means you get a longer step with every stride, without having to over-reach or over stride (more on this later). In other words, you go farther, without additional effort.

Try it sometime on a treadmill for kicks. Run at 5 miles an hour and check out your stride. Now go up on your toes without increasing your effort. Put your finger over the *quickfast* button because, chances are, you'll have to jump up the speed on the treadmill or you'll run right off it. With the same effort, you go farther with each stride when you're on your toes. Just one more reason it's no wonder toe runners are breaking all the world records out there.

Running barefoot is all about running on your toes. Strike your heel once, and you go home.

7 Expectations for New Barefoot Runners

While I'm asking you to let go of outcome, it's still natural for you to wonder about what you should expect so you know you're on the right track. Here are 7 common situations you may experience during the early transition phase.

1. **The Ground Will Feel Hard.** This is to be expected! You have baby soft feet when you start out, and it takes time for your feet to adjust to the new surfaces. But, rest assured, that no matter how baby soft your feet feel now, they will adapt to the point where you'll find yourself welcoming the small pebbles beneath your feet.

2. **In the Beginning, Your Skin Will Often Feel Tender.** If you run or walk every other day (or even a little less often), you'll be giving your skin a chance to grow back stronger than ever before. Expect your skin to cycle with your runs, between feeling strong, then tender, then stronger yet again.

3. **You May Experience Blisters.** I hope you'll stop before the hot spots on the bottom of your feet develop into blisters. But it's likely you might be having too much fun to want to stop in time!

4. **Your Arches and Calves Will Fatigue.** Don't be surprised if the following day your feet and calves feel sore, as if you've squashed your feet and done hundreds of calf raises. It's just your muscles' way of saying, "Hi, we're still here and ready to start working again!"

5. **With Time, You May Need to Invest in an Extra Wide Shoe.** Your forefeet will grow wider as your toes learn to grab and feel the ground. This is a great thing. A wider platform provides more stability and shock absorption than a narrow platform, which means you'll be less likely to roll an ankle.

6. **You'll Learn a New Stride.** You'll learn you have to stand tall to keep your

core engaged and to land on your toes. Land light and listen. If you're slapping the ground hard, get forward on your forefoot. If you're pitter-pattering light, you're doing it right!

7. **Everything Under the Skin Will Fatigue and Then Grow Strong.** It takes time. Listen to your feet and in particular your skin. Jumping straight to minimalist shoes can trick you if you don't start slowly.

Consider starting truly barefoot and going barefoot every other day at most. In between, you can rest your feet in your old supportive shoes, orthotics, or insoles (more on this in the chapter on footwear). Just make sure you do your workouts barefoot. When you go sans shoes, it's hard to go too far. When the skin gets sore, you know it's time to go home. In this game, it's all about awareness: awareness of yourself and awareness of the ground. Learn to be aware, and you'll learn to fly!

Exercise: The Barefoot Strike

I like using this demonstration that Barefoot Ted shared at one of our clinics.

Try this: When you're wearing shoes, you tend to land flat-footed or on your heels. Try standing upright, then stomping one foot into the ground directly beneath you and notice what that feels like. Feel the force? This simulates a midfoot strike. Repeat it a few times with your eyes closed and feel the impact and where it travels through your body.

If you desire, you can stomp that same foot onto the ground on your heel, but that puts so much force on you, I can't recommend it. This action simulates a heel strike. Even in your most cushioned shoe, that force travels straight up through your body.

Now put your foot out in front of you about a foot and stomp down on the ground on your toes. It's difficult trying to stomp on your forefoot, isn't it? This is how you run barefoot. Notice any difference? Try closing your eyes and feel the force this time.

You'll see there's far less force carried through your toes and ball of your foot into your body than if you stomp flat-footed on the ground right beneath you. And that's the whole point of barefoot running. We're not growing stronger knees (though they will get healthier), and we're not building shock-resistant bodies. Instead, we're learning a way to avoid the shock in the first place. We're learning to run soft and light as a feather.

Watch ballet dancers on their toes, watch them also land from a jump. They move and land lightly. When we're running barefoot, we're not absorbing the shock, we're moving light and using it for our springs. Using shock for propulsion is faster and more efficient.

Practice this drill a few times to see what I mean, then show it to your friends and see their response as well.

A Short Barefoot Stride vs. a Long Shod Stride

When you're barefoot, you tend to land with your feet and legs relatively close to your body, with a short stride. To go faster, you simply increase the number of strides you take per minute, rather than lengthening the distance you take per stride.

With a somewhat heavy running shoe on, it's difficult to increase the number of strides you take per minute. Instead, with the heavy rubberized heel on a running shoe, it becomes easy to over stride.

When you land barefoot, your lower leg never goes past perpendicular with the

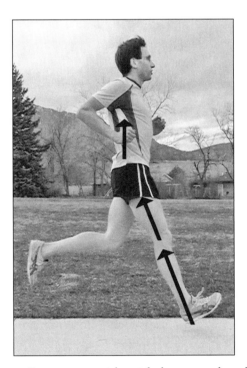 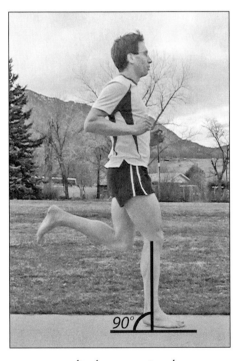

Runner over strides with shoes on and reaches past perpendicular—creating dangerous deceleration forces with each landing. After years of running light, I had great difficulty and some fear in getting my body to stride out and land on my heels for this photo.

ground. Why? Because going farther would generate immediate pain through the foot and up the leg—like you, I don't like pain, and when I'm running barefoot, I'm aware of pain and force with each and every stride.

But in a shoe, you can extend the leg past perpendicular with the ground. In fact, with a heavily cushioned heel, your shoes promote this kind of a stride. The challenge is this: when you're out past perpendicular, or what I refer to as "90 degrees," you lock out your natural shock-absorbing mechanism. No longer can you use your foot, arch, Achilles, calf, and more as it was designed, but instead the force travels straight up through your body.

●°°₀ FOOT NOTE

Have you ever watched videos of Abebe Bikila winning the marathon in the 1960 Olympics in Rome? He did it barefoot and with tiny, short strides.

He was sponsored by Adidas, but the day before the Olympics, he discovered the shoes Adidas sent him were too small. Luckily, he had grown up barefoot in Africa and still continued to train barefoot. Thus, he decided to run the race entirely without shoes.

It turns out with the smooth early roads and a nighttime finish on cobblestones, barefoot running actually gave Abebe an advantage over his competition. It helped him keep a short, efficient stride on the smooth roads. Then, in the dark, he was guided along the cobblestones with his extrasensory bare feet while his competition only had sight to rely on.

Most importantly for this discussion, if you see Abebe Bikila running barefoot in the 1960 Olympics, he does it with nice short strides—his legs never extending past perpendicular or 90 degrees. And then if you watch him in 1964, now sponsored by Tiger, later known as Asics, as he races along in shoes, he's reaching out with his leg past perpendicular. This is a telltale sign of what's to come, and though he won the 1964 Olympics, he was plagued with stress fractures thereafter.

Why? Because once you go past the 90-degree mark, it doesn't matter how strong you are, where you come from, your magical running past, the strength of your feet, or the shock absorption in your shoes. Once you pass 90 degrees, you've locked out the natural shock-absorbing mechanism of your feet and legs, and you're now sending the shock straight up your body.

In this case, overextending or what is referred to as striding out even minutely punished his legs, forcing the impact to travel up through his body, rather than be absorbed and rebounded with each stride. Over time striding out gets even the best of us.

While a longer stride seems efficient in the moment, and, admittedly, Bikila was faster by 3 minutes in shoes (though it may have been the course), it takes one heck of a toll on the body. Not just in terms of shock, but in terms of sheer workload too. Biomechanically, when you over stride, or extend past perpendicular, your foot acts as a brake with each stride.

In other words, you decelerate your foot, leg, and body each time you make contact with the ground; so you strike and slow down, and then must reaccelerate the leg with each push-off. This means you're doing double the work you have to. When you land short, with or without a shoe, your foot and leg act as a wheel, rolling along without loss of speed. And landing short, your foot acts as a spring, absorbing shock, then rebounding at the end of each stride. Short barefoot strides are far more efficient.

When you're running barefoot, you're running like a cookie thief, stealing into the kitchen at night. You're nice and light, up on your tippy toes, trying to make as little noise or, in this case, impact as possible.

Let's take a look at another world-class champion, Haile Gebrselassie, who also grew up running barefoot. He still runs with this short, efficient stride, yet with incredible turnover. He's only 5 feet 4 inches tall, immediately blowing away the stereotype of a tall African distance runner. You might think he would try to compensate by overextending his stride. In fact, he does the opposite. He keeps his stride extra short, stays high on his toes, and concentrates on incredibly fast leg turnovers with a remarkable 180 to 190 strides per minute.

When running barefoot, we're emulating Haile and aiming for high turnover speed, with a short stride. Keep the strides short, keep your shock absorber engaged, and keep yourself efficient.

Picture this analogy. A short stride is like riding your bike in an easier gear. It rests your legs more, letting your lungs and heart do more of the work. This technique keeps you from fatigue, letting you go farther and faster before your legs give out.

◐°∘°₀ FOOT NOTE

First and Second Gear

One way to look at the foot and leg is as a 2-speed bicycle. When you're in first gear, you're walking or rolling from your heel to your toe. This gives you great stability, though it barely engages both your forefoot springs and your Achilles. But as you move forward, you stride like a wheel, rolling from heel to toe, spending most of the time rolling off your forefoot.

Now when you're running on your forefoot, it's like you're in second gear. You're no longer locked in at the heel. You've gone from a 1-speed, with your leg as a lever, to a 2-speed, with your leg and foot as two levers. You've doubled the leverage, increased your stride length without overextending your legs, and you're loading both the midfoot with energy and, especially, that incredibly strong and elastic Achilles.

When you're on your heel, you're locked in first; but on your toes, you've got one heck of a faster second gear. That's why all sprinting is done on our toes! And long-distance running would be too, if our shoes didn't force us onto our heels, and we built up our Achilles strength slowly. (Unfortunately, having spent the majority of our lives in traditional running shoes our Achilles and calves are incredibly weak. Trying to run long distances on our toes without an incredibly gradual increase would result in muscle or tendon strains or bad tears.)

Exercise: Paddle Along

Here's a fun imagery exercise to help you get used to the feeling of turning your feet over more quickly.

Try this: As you're running along, picture your legs and feet as a giant paddle-wheel. They rotate forward, catching the water, grabbing as much of it as they can, then dumping it out behind them.

Pretend your feet are paddles and catch the ground as you land. Then pull up on your feet, getting them up and out of the water as fast as possible. Bring your heels up high as you pull out of the water and up to your butt behind you.

Think of the paddlewheel below and slightly in front of you. When your foot lifts off the ground, think of it as trying to bring your foot back underneath your body, rather than behind you.

Be the paddlewheel and keep the strides short, turn the feet around fast, and have some fun!

Think, also, of running on hot coals. If you're running on hot coals, you're hitting the ground and bringing the feet back up almost instantly, or as fast as possible. This has you staying on the ground for the least amount of time you can.

Running Light Means Running Quiet

Lao Tzu said, "A good runner leaves no footprints." As a barefoot runner, I add, "A good runner makes no sound."

You can learn a lot by listening to a runner striking the ground. Great runners are

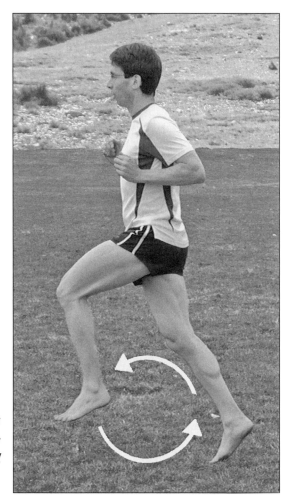

Paddlewheel drill: Bring your legs around in front of you as if they're a spinning riverboat paddlewheel moving through the water.

quiet. Barefoot runners are nearly silent. The quieter you are, the softer you meet the ground. After some practice, you'll be surprised at how often you'll startle people who won't hear you coming.

Sakai, a Marathon Monk from Mount Hiei in Japan, was asked what frightened him most during his runs in the woods. Was it darkness? Wild animals? Apparitions? He said, "People! They think I am a ghost and let out terrible screams."

Running light is an essential skill for barefoot running. When you run light, you put less pressure on your joints and muscles. Running light saves everything and allows you to run longer with less effort.

Exercise: Running Quiet

Try this: Imagine you're as light as a feather and that a silvery string is pulling you up through your head and into the sky. Stare at a star, or up at the sky, feel yourself get lighter with each breath, picture yourself weightless, and envision your feet floating above the ground.

When it comes time to start barefoot running, practice light runs. Head out with the idea in mind of running with the least impact possible, keeping your feet out in front of you, and absorbing shock with your muscles, not your joints. Keep your arms up high and listen to the sound your feet make on impact. The more you stay on the balls of your feet, the lighter you run, and the quieter you'll be. Noise is force, and noise is impact. Stay on the balls of your feet and go light. How silent can you be?

Get good at this, and over time you'll not only be light on your feet, but you'll find yourself going farther and faster than ever before because light is efficient. The less work you have to do to raise or lower the body, the more work can go into moving you forward. Get light, and you'll find you can run mile after mile, hour after hour, floating above the terrain, almost effortlessly.

Be the Humble Barefoot Runner

As barefoot running takes off and becomes more accepted by mainstream America, we'll see people succeed beyond their wildest dreams and others who turn away injured. The number one way to ensure you don't fall into the latter category is by practicing humility.

As I'm always apt to say, we're turning everything on its head with barefoot running. Many things that you learned from high school coaches, running partners, and shoe salesmen over the years may not be true, such as these maxims we've turned upside down:

#1 Pain equals gain. *False.*

#2 The harder you work, the faster you reap benefits. *False.*

#3 Taking time off means you're lazy. *False.*

You need to be willing to wipe the slate clean and admit that you may not know everything about running. This is the best advice I can give for staying injury-free.

Maybe you've believed you were born as a heel striker. Maybe you've believed the longer your stride, the faster and farther you would go. So it may take a combination of humility, a barefooted leap of faith, and some pretty big paradigm shifts to learn a completely new way of running that is not only kinder on your body, but allows you to be lighter, faster, and more aware of your body, the earth, and those around you.

As one of my students, Scott McLean, always says, "Barefoot running is running without pride!"

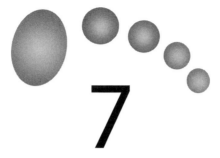

7

Turn Your Feet into Living Shoes

The human foot is a masterpiece of engineering and a work of art.
—Leonardo da Vinci

To build your feet stronger, it helps tremendously to understand what the foot really is, its integral parts, and these parts work together so you can build your strongest feet ever.

Many of us runners have been told how weak our feet are, and how they're not meant to handle the "abuse" of running. The reality is they're not the limp models you've been shown in doctor's offices, which collapse with the slightest touch. Instead, they're incredible massive springs that are meant to coil and recoil with every single step. They're also dynamic—able to handle different contours, surfaces, speeds, and angles, all in an instant. They house thousands of nerve endings that enable sense or feel for the ground, giving us fantastic balance and the ability to handle challenging three-dimensional surfaces.

There's nothing in the mechanical world that matches the sophistication, complexity, and multi-tasking ability of the foot. Just look at robots. The most sophisticated humanoid robots are equipped with the same flat one-segmented, boot-like "feet" used decades ago, precisely due to the fact that the human foot is one of the most complicated body parts in regard to bones, muscles, and nerves.

The Importance of Strengthening Your Feet

If you want to run better, have fewer aches and pains, or be healthier and happier in general, then you need strong, healthy, happy feet—not just for running, but for every activity in your life.

Did you know the average 150-pound person puts 2,000 tons of cumulative weight on his or her feet, every single day? That's not through running. That's just getting around. Even if you never ran a day in your life, you're likely to get back, hip, neck, and other injuries if you never strengthen your feet.

Even with today's super high-tech shoes, injuries are on the increase. According to the American Academy of Orthopedic Surgeons, in 2006, one out of six people or 43.1 million Americans suffered foot ailments.

Among cultures that don't wear shoes, approximately 2 percent of the population has foot-related injuries, compared to 70 percent among shoe-wearing societies. And people wearing shoes have feet at least 40 to 50 percent weaker than in shoeless populations. In other words, the average American's foot is only half as strong as it should be.

As we've so often heard, perception dictates reality. If we think of the feet as weak and fragile, then we end up with weak and fragile feet. We also think of them as immovable, unbendable stubs that we need to stuff in shoes for protection. But our feet aren't fragile, and far from unbendable. They're dynamic, changing, multi-piece, multi-sensory devices—that is, until we stuff them in shoes. It's in a shoe that perception becomes reality. In a shoe, our feet lose the ability to sense, adjust, adapt, flex, and stay strong and become those weakened, inflexible stubs we need to protect.

According to evolutionary biologists, it's our magnificent two feet that helped us evolve into the amazing species we are today. The foot made us who we are, made us strong, light, smart, and agile, and helped us to run, thrive, and survive.

In this chapter we'll look at this magnificent marvel, help you understand how it works and why, and then how to build your strongest feet ever. We will dig deep inside, looking at the structure of the foot and the physics behind its design.

And Now ... the Foot

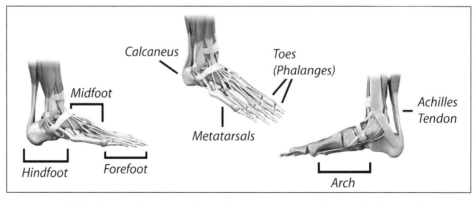

A remarkable design of nature, when allowed to work and move freely, the foot provides strength, stability, and amazing shock absorption.

We'll start from the inside out and look at the inner workings of this marvel. Since this isn't a high school biology class, we'll just briefly cover the basics, starting from the inside out, and head to specific parts of the foot.

FOOT NOTE

Helpful Terms to Know

Bones: Your feet have over one quarter of all of the bones in the human body, 56 in all. The foot has 28 bones, 26 that most people count, and 2 little ones, called sesamoid bones, under the big toe's joint, which protect its large tendon. Each bone has its own unique purpose and design. There are 14 toe bones which grab, 5 midfoot metatarsals which act as springs, and 7 bones of the hindfoot or heel, which help support weight and hold everything together.

Consider the bones the foundation of the foot. They're both what hold it together and help turn it into a spring.

Joints: All bones connect or hinge at joints. There are 37 different joints in the foot.

Ligaments: There are 107 ligaments that crisscross the joints in the foot. They're semi-elastic fibers that help the joints move at hinges. Since they stretch a bit, they allow the joints to expand or open up a bit when you move, helping with shock absorption and handling weight.

Cartilage: Resilient connective tissue covers and connects bones providing cushioning and protecting against shock.

Muscles: There are 19 different muscles of the foot. Each pulls on an individual tendon that attaches to a bone to provide support and move joints.

Tendons: Each foot has 19 tendons—highly elastic fibers that connect muscles to joints. Each muscle has a connecting tendon. This is where the majority of the energy is stored in the foot, as tendons can store and return up to 93 percent of the energy they receive.

Sweat Glands: Your foot has over 250,000 sweat glands, capable of producing over a half pint of sweat from each foot daily (an important reason to wear breathable footwear!).

Plantar Fascia: A broad span of ligament-like tissue fans out across the sole, covering the foot from the forefoot to the heel. It helps hold the foot together and provides cushioning.

These 3 main sections of the foot work together:

1. **Midfoot**—made up of slightly bow-shaped bones, called metatarsals, which help absorb energy

2. **Forefoot**—comprised of toes and joints that grab

3. **Hindfoot**—made up of the largest bones of the foot that help with weight-bearing and providing stability

The midfoot bridges

One way to view the foot is as a living, breathing bridge. It absorbs energy, returns it, and despite a heavy load, or strong winds, always returns back to center. In the case of the foot, you can think of it as a two-level bridge. Above is a high-tensioned suspension bridge and, below, a giant stone arch.

The 5 metatarsals of the foot and their ligaments, tendons, and connective tissue act as giant energy storage devices and shock-absorbers. They're held together under tension, and when you add weight, they get even tighter. Step down, and your midfoot stores energy. Step up, it snaps or springs right back into place again.

The metatarsals are also special because each one can move independently of the other, allowing the foot to change shape and mold with the terrain. This helps you keep your balance and stability even on the harshest of terrain. (That is, unless you keep your foot in a shoe, in which case you lose all of this midfoot flexibility and strength. In essence, you lock out your adaptable spring, which hinders your ability to absorb impact and handle uneven terrain.)

Beneath the metatarsals are two giant arches. There's one stretching the length of the foot, and one stretching the width of the foot. An arch is defined as a weight-bearing structure that gets *stronger* under load. This is particularly important, because your arches don't collapse under weight as you've likely been told, but instead get stronger and then rebound. Trouble is, if you don't strengthen the muscles that hold the arches up, they become atrophied. Once this occurs, the connective tissue, commonly plantar fascia, is forced to hold the arches up. Since plantar fascia were never intended to do the work of muscles, they become stressed, strained, inflamed, or torn. And voila! You have a recipe for plantar fasciitis.

If you keep your muscles strong, however, the suspension bridge above and the arches below will take almost all of the force you give it on landing, and return it right back (rebound). In essence, your foot can turn gravity into forward momentum. What an incredibly efficient device!

A note about arches and bridge design. Stone arches work fantastic under compression, but don't do well with twisting, pulling, or sheering. Human bones work just the same way. They're one fifth the weight of steel, but can handle twice the compression force of granite and 4 times the force of concrete. However, just like granite and concrete, human bones can't handle sheering, pulling, or torsion forces, the *exact* forces amplified by most shoes.

Imagine the muscles in your feet as the strings of a marionette. When your feet are weak, it's as if your muscles are as limp as the strings of the marionette. But when you pull up on the strings, such as with strong, healthy foot muscles, the marionette springs to life and takes form.

Look at your foot, lift your toes, then curl them again. As you flex things, can you see the cables of your foot (your muscles, tendons, and to a lesser extent your ligaments) tighten and release? Your foot is a series of cables or wires working in harmony under tension. In combination with your arch, these cables work to absorb energy when you land or step down, and rebound this energy when you lift off the ground.

The forefoot anchor

For a bridge to be strong, it needs support at both ends. This helps anchor the arches and tie in the cables of your suspension bridges, known as your feet. The two ends of your bridges are your toes and your heels. The small bones of the toes (3 in each small toe, 2 in the big toe) connect to 18 of the 19 muscles in your feet. This is important as strong toes strengthen and hold together your entire foot.

Few people realize that when you run, your toes should be active. Barefoot, you pull up your toes (dorsiflexion) before striking the ground, preloading the arch, and upon impact, your toes push down (plantar flexion) grabbing the ground and bracing the arch. When you work your toes, you strengthen your arch and your entire foot. Conversely, when your toes are weak, your entire foot is weak. This is exceptionally important, because in almost all modern running shoes your toes are eliminated from your stride. Toe-spring, the upward curvature found at the front of shoes, keeps your toes off the ground, while stiff shoes further prohibit your toes from experiencing a full range of motion.

A last thought on the toes. Your toes naturally spread. If you look at the toes of someone who's been barefoot an entire lifetime, you'll see a natural large gap between the big toe and the second toe. The more your toes spread, the wider your forefoot, the greater your stability when you stand, walk, or run, and the more you spread out the impact.

Picture a narrow foot and a wide foot as the difference between sinking through snow in a regular shoe and staying afloat in a snowshoe. When your toes can spread, you have a bigger paddle for propulsion, balance, and weight distribution, keeping you from harm.

Unfortunately, when you're in a shoe, your toes are bound in a very narrow passageway, keeping them from spreading and, over time, changing your feet to where your first and fifth toes tend to point inward. By keeping your feet from spreading, you're not only losing surface area for balance and stability, but forcing tremendous pressure onto a very small part of the foot.

The hindfoot anchor

At the other end of your bridge are the 7 big bones of the foot, all intricately wedged together like fine masonry work. These bones have the ability to rotate the entire foot slightly inward like a screw. The left foot rotates inward toward the right, and the right foot rotates inward toward the left. Despite this flexibility, these bones have limited overall mobility to anchor the foot and bear a heavy weight.

When you're a hunter carrying food home, you're walking on your heels. And if you're on the edge of a rocky slope, you've got your heels firmly planted into the ground. These 7 bones give your feet great strength and stability. What they do *not* do is store energy. That's the combined job of your forefoot and midfoot. And that's important because when you land on your heel, you're not taking advantage of your foot's natural springs.

If the midfoot and arch creates the first spring, the second spring in your natural shock-absorption system is your Achilles tendon—the strongest, most resilient, and elastic tendon in your body. Your Achilles tendon connects your calf to your heel and can handle nearly a ton of weight. The Achilles is essential for efficient running and forward propulsion. Unfortunately, when you land on your heels, you lock out almost all of its abilities.

Our feet work great because each part is allowed to move independently, and everything works together to move and adapt to the terrain and to coil like a spring. Each part of the foot is integral to the whole, and each has its own independent job. Yet when you put that foot in a shoe, you turn a multi-segmented, dynamic, spring-loaded device into a solid piece of wood.

In running, you load your foot, or land down on it, then you lift up. Voila, the coil spring returns, rebounding you forward, and returning almost all of the energy it absorbed into forward momentum. When you absorb impact, these actions occur at once:

- Compress your arches
- Stretch the tendons on each muscle that connect your toes to your foot
- Stretch the Achilles tendon, connecting the foot to the calf
- Compress your cartilage, which acts as a bumper by each joint
- Stretch your ligaments, which let the joints spread and absorb shock
- Stretch your plantar fascia, taking its wavy bundles of fibers, pulling them taut and long

Your foot is a magnificent piece of machinery, and quite the incredible spring. The trick is, it only works if you promote its strength and flexibility, allow it to move freely, and, in particular, allow natural motion of the toes.

Try the following foot exercises to strengthen and condition your feet for barefoot running.

Warm-up Exercises

Though I've taught a lot of ball exercises, and thought I'd tried just about all of them under the sun, this unique sequence of exercises comes from Pat Guyton and Jan Dunn, who teach the Eric Franklin conditioning method (www.franklinmethodtrain ing.com) along with Pilates for rehabilitation and dancing. It's a great way to warm up the feet, get the muscles firing, and help train the connection between your mind and feet.

In short, the following exercises, all of which can be done on their own or as part of this warm-up series, do 4 key things:

1. Warm up foot muscles

2. Stretch out the foot

3. Strengthen foot muscles

4. Establish a kinesthetic loop between your brain and your foot

In essence, these exercises help wake up the neurological connection between foot and brain, essential for strength, movement, coordination, and balance.

Step 1—Loosen Up. Obtain a small inflatable ball, just bigger than a tennis ball (we use the Eric Franklin 10 cm textured Franklin balls and 10 cm smooth Franklin balls and equivalent Yamuna or RunBare balls). Begin by moving the arch of your foot back and forth across the ball for a minute. You don't need to bend or move your knee to do this. Just roll your foot.

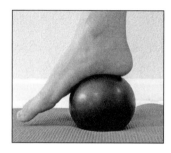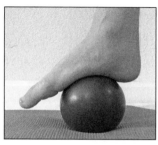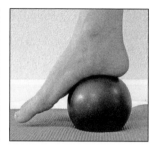

Rolling your foot back and forth on a ball helps wake up the nerves and muscles of your feet.

Step 2—Stretch Out Your Mets (Metatarsals). After a minute, begin moving your forefoot from side to side over the ball, move it down to one side, and then back down to the other, repeating 5 times. This is also a great exercise for building flexibility in the forefoot as it relaxes and stretches the ligaments and tendons between your metatarsals, important for keeping your feet supple and healthy, particularly when running on uneven terrain.

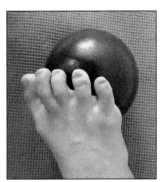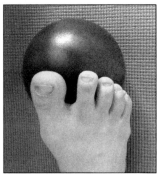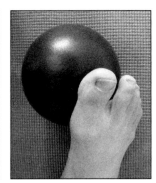

Wake up your metatarsals by rolling your forefoot sideways and down while hugging the sides of the ball. Roll down one side, then back up and down the other.

Step 3—Wake Up Your Dorsiflexors. After you've awakened and stretched out your metatarsals, continue rolling your forefoot slowly sideways across the top of the ball, but this time raise up your foot as you raise up your toes. This is the reverse of the previous exercise. Repeat this for a set of 5 to each side as well. This helps reawaken the flexibility and strength of the extensors in your toes, which is particularly important for preloading your arch and keeping your toes above the ground (before impact) when barefoot running (in other words, you'll prevent toe stubbing).

Step 4—Get Jiggy with the Heels. Next roll your foot forward on the ball until your forefoot's on the ground and your heel is on the ball. Then roll your heel side to side over the ball, repeating 5 times. Again you don't have to flex or move your knee. All movement should come from the foot. This helps awaken rotational control of the foot, something that's dormant in a shoe.

Step 5—Say Hello to Your Toes. Next, roll your heel back and put your toes on top of the ball. Grab and dig into the ball with your toes for one minute, grabbing and releasing.

Step 6—Balancing on the Balls. With all of the core strength work I recommend for barefoot running, this is a personal favorite of mine. It helps with coordination, balance, and strength of the foot, and if you get good at this, you can use it for core strength as well. For the next minute, practice standing on one ball, with the other leg suspended, with it placed beneath your arch, or slightly forward onto your forefoot.

Stand and hold for a few seconds, recover and repeat, for up to one minute.

Gone Skiing. There's one more foot warm-up exercise we found particularly challenging and enjoyable. It's best to do this one where you have a partner or something to hold onto to keep from falling. You want to stand on two balls, with one under the arch of each foot. Next, roll backward on both balls onto your forefeet, then forward onto your heels.

This is best practiced while holding onto something or someone at first. Roll back and forth for one minute to begin. Over time, work on having less and less support for balance, instead letting your feet and core do the work. This exercise helps build the connection between your mind and your feet, while working all of your stabilizing muscles.

Before we get into the strengthening exercises, I have another personal favorite warm-up exercise you may already be familiar with:

Foot Circles. With your leg extended on a bench, rotate your foot counter clockwise for 10 circles without moving your leg. Then reverse direction for another count of 10.

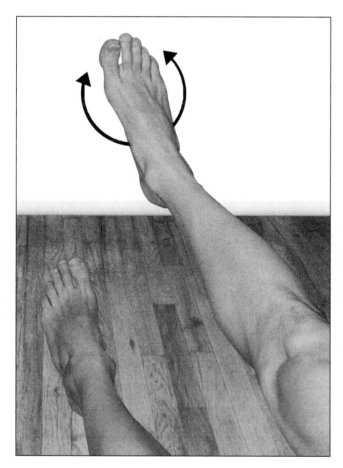

Draw circles with your feet, moving only from the ankles (your feet should not move). For an advanced version, draw out the letters of the alphabet!

Strengthening Exercises

This next section describes some fantastic exercises for building foot strength, coordination, balance and flexibility. *Grabbing Exercises* can be practiced daily over time. However, more intense exercises, such as *Raising Exercises*, *Resistance/Band Exercises*, and *Toe Movement Exercises* should be practiced, at most, every other day, just like lifting weights.

Remember, you build muscle by stressing the fibers and building them back stronger. Because of this process, you never want to work muscles that are still sore; you won't make them stronger, but simply delay recovery at best, or tear muscles at worst.

FOOT NOTE

DOMS, or Delayed Onset Muscle Soreness is muscle soreness on the second and third days, particularly following the start of a new exercise, movement, or exercise program. It's common when you begin to prepare for barefoot running because you are essentially creating microscopic tears to the muscles, which take time to heal. It's not something to worry about; however, never repeat the offending exercise that made you sore until you're 100 percent recovered. Otherwise, you'll delay recovery or could potentially end up tearing your muscles apart.

Grabbing exercises

By strengthening the toes, you strengthen the entire foot and help build healthy arches. These exercises are a great way to warm up before a barefoot jog or run and help sustain healthy circulation levels in your lower legs and feet while sitting at a desk or on a plane.

- **The Golf Ball Grab.** This is one of the best exercises for your feet. It helps strengthen your feet and toes, build flexibility, and widen your forefoot, promoting a nice spread between your big toe and your second toe.

  Simply grab a golf ball with your toes. Hold for 5 or 10 seconds, then repeat. Do a set of 10 to 20 grabs your first time, then build up from there.

  As we've seen, almost every muscle of your foot attaches to your toes. By grabbing a ball, you're working nearly every muscle of the foot, and in particular, you're waking up and strengthening your long-dormant arch.

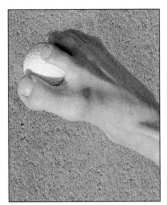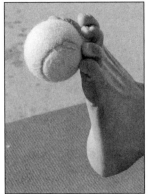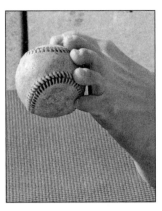

Golf Ball Grab: Strengthen your feet by working to grab a golf ball. Jessica has worked her way up to tennis balls and now baseballs gaining tremendous dexterity, flexibility, and strength.

Variations: If you get really good, you can try picking up the ball, passing it from foot to foot, and even work up to larger balls, such as tennis balls and baseballs. Try walking around your house holding golf balls with your feet, or do a Pilates or balance routine without letting go of a ball. Want to work on toe coordination? Consider lifting marbles as well. Try to lift them between each individual toe, rather than just with your big toe.

- **Towel Scrunch.** This is a simpler version of the golf ball grab. Simply roll up a towel, place it beneath your feet, and grab it with your toes. Again hold for 5 to 10 seconds, then repeat for a set of 10.

- **Desk Grab.** When you find yourself stuck at a desk for hours at a time, try grabbing the desktop or legs of the desk with your feet. Hold for a count of 5 to 10 seconds. Then release. Or keep a golf ball under your desk, kick off your shoes, and strengthen those toes while no one is looking.

- **Inch Worm.** This is a more dynamic version of a scrunch or grab. It's easier to do this sitting rather than standing when you first begin. Grab the ground (any surface will work) and pull your foot forward and repeat, inch worming along, until it's extended out in front of you. Then reverse directions and push your foot back with your toes. You may not be used to moving your toes this way; however, this aids with dorsiflexion (lifting up) with your toes, critical for a good stride.

- **Tiger Walk.** We use this exercise at almost all beginner clinics and it is covered in more detail in an earlier chapter. However, walk with your weight slightly on your forefoot and your heel just off the ground as you visualize yourself with cat claws. Grab the ground and pull yourself forward with each and every step. Start with 50 to 100 yards of this exercise, then increase your distance over time. This can be done on any surface; the coarser the surface, the more it'll help with pad development as well.

- **Stick Game.** You may have read about the ball games used by the Tarahumara in Christopher McDougall's *Born to Run*. This is a variation of a common Native American game practiced for thousands of years. Teams race while kicking an 8- to 10-inch by 1-inch diameter stick to the finish line. Grabbing and kicking the stick forces you to work all the muscles of your foot, both for grabbing (plantar flexion) and for extending (dorsiflexion).

  Attempt to kick a small stick from one end of a park to the other, or better yet, bring along your barefooted friends and make a game of it! Warning, this exercise does a great job of strengthening the foot, but will also scuff up the top of your toes. However, this is fantastic for strengthening the top skin of your foot, which is important if you plan on running rocky trails barefoot.

Raising exercises

- **Lifting Your Arch.** While standing with your foot planted firmly on the ground, imagine a string pulling through your arch and through the top of your feet. Lift your arch to the sky without moving your toes. Imagine your arch as a bridge that grows taller with each upward pull. Hold for a count of 5 and repeat for a total of 10 times to begin.

The next 3 exercises are commonly referred to as calf raises. While they do have the benefit of strengthening your calves and Achilles, they require firing of nearly every muscle of the foot and ankle to do so, building foot strength, coordination, and balance.

- **Straight Toe Stands.** Standing in front of a mirror with both feet pointed in front of you (shoulder width apart), slowly raise yourself onto your toes, then lower your feet back down. Do this on a 5 count to begin, 2 seconds to raise your feet, and 3 to lower them. Concentrate on control over speed, going slowly and stopping just shy of your heels hitting the ground. Repeat for a set of 10 to begin.

  Over time you can progress to 3 sets, then begin doing this exercise with one leg at a time. However, make sure you have your balance first—engage your core and make sure you do the exercise *without* holding on to the mirror or anything else. Too difficult in the beginning? Then hold on lightly, but keep yourself tall and straight. If you're gripping too hard, you'll negate the benefits for your feet.

A note of caution here, when you begin barefoot running, your calves are much weaker than you think. Even if this exercise feels easy, only do one set to begin. Your calves will likely be sore the next day, and perhaps a bit more sore the following day.

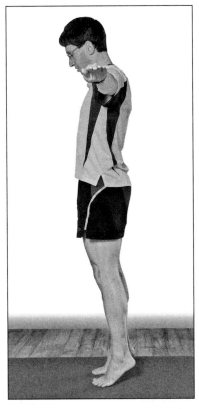

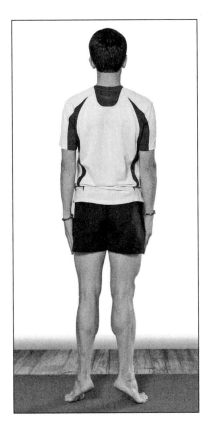

Slow, controlled calf raises with your arms extended give you greater muscle and balance co-ordination while strengthening your core.

Outer Toe Stands

- **Outer Toe Stands.** Stand with your toes pointed outward and your heels slightly touching. Slowly raise yourself onto your toes so that your heels are no longer in contact with each other. Lower your feet back to your starting position. Repeat for no more than a set of 10 for your first time, and then build into multiple sets. Make sure you engage your core, stand tall (remember the silvery string), and again do not hold on to anything else. Like the previous exercise, this is best practiced in front of a mirror.

- **Inner Toe Stands.** Similar to both previous exercises, however, point your toes inward to where they almost touch before you stand. This one may feel particularly awkward and off-balance in the beginning. This exercise is a bit awkward, therefore, holding onto something for a little support is okay in the beginning, as long as you stand upright. Repeat for 10 repetitions to begin.

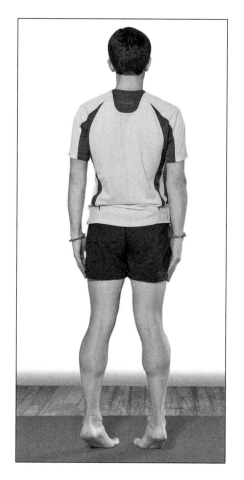

Inner Toe Stands

Resistance/band exercises

These exercises can be done with physical therapy bands such as Therabands (different colors for different resistance levels), the RubberBanditz, or even cut up old inner tubes. Start with very little resistance to begin. Build up your number of sets, and then begin increasing resistance.

- **Pulling In.** With the band directly in front of you, dorsiflex your foot (bring your forefoot toward you). This should also be done on a 3 count and repeated for a set of 10.

- **Rotating In.** Sit on the floor with your legs stretched out in front of you. Affix one end of a band to an object directly to your side and place the other end around your foot near the ball of the foot (up high, but where it won't slip off your foot). (For the left foot, keep the band to your left side, reverse for your right.) With the band looped around near the ball of your foot, gently and slowly rotate your foot inward while pivoting on your heel. Keep your leg on the ground and make sure there is no leg movement. This may feel awkward or jerky at first. Do the rotation on a 3 count, one second to rotate in, two seconds to rotate back out. Repeat for a set of 10.

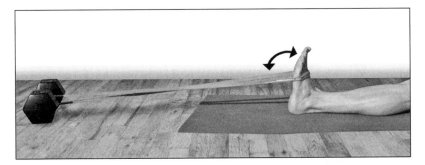

Make sure the band or belt won't slip off your foot, then gently pull your foot up and toward you while keeping your heel on the ground.

- **Rotating Out.** Repeat the same exercise but with the band and direction reversed. For your left side, place the band directly to the right of you, and vice versa. Here, slowly rotate your foot outward while pivoting on your heel, again with your leg on the ground and without leg movement. Repeat for a set of 10.

- **Alphabet (with or without resistance).** This should be done without resistance to begin, and then over time can be done with a resistance band of your choice. Keep your foot in front of you with your heel 2–3 inches above the ground. Using your forefoot, draw out the individual letters of the alphabet. Make sure you do not draw the alphabet with your leg. This is a foot and ankle exercise only.

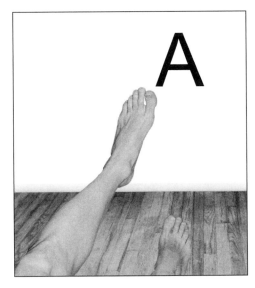

Draw out the letters of the alphabet with your resistance band or belt secured around your foot. Make sure you do not move your leg, only your foot and ankle.

Toe movement exercises

People who are born without arms, or have impaired arm ability, often turn to their feet to do almost every daily skill others do with their hands. Our feet are capable of holding, writing, painting, cooking, even turning door knobs and more, if we work on it diligently.

For these exercises, we must reawaken the coordination and movement of each individual toe. This can be challenging and take quite a bit of time and dedication. Start slowly and be patient.

- **Raising Toes.** This is the simplest one of the bunch. You want to be seated during this exercise with your foot firmly planted on the ground. From here raise your toes away from the floor and hold for a count of 5. Repeat for a set of 10. As an advanced exercise, work on raising each toe individually, fanning out from your biggest toe to your smallest.

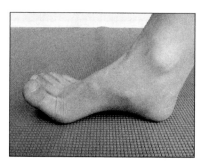 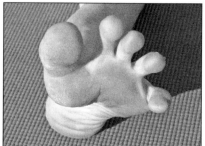

Raise your toes with your feet on the floor. Hold for a count of 5, then repeat.

Toe Spread: Work to spread your toes. Be patient, this one's mentally challenging.

- **Toe Spread.** Working to spread your toes may be a difficult task, particularly if your feet have been squashed in shoes for years. While keeping your heels on the ground, work to bring your toes apart as far as possible. At first you may only be able to visualize your toes spreading or moving apart in your head. Give it time. Attempt to hold your toes apart for a count of 5. Repeat for up to 10 times.

- **Tapping Keys.** Pretend your toes are your fingers, and you're playing the piano. With your heel firmly on the ground, raise and lower each toe individually from your biggest to your smallest. You may have to visualize this in your head for many practice sessions before you can do it, but keep working at it, and you may amaze yourself! Chopsticks, anyone?

From here, see what other activities your feet and toes can do. Personally, I like picking things up with my feet instead of reaching down. It strengthens all muscles of the feet and is fun, not to mention easier than bending down, once you get the hang of it!

Many great devices can help build foot strength and flexibility too. Among my favorites are YogaToes—a device you slip on your foot that helps spread your toes (it's like the toe spreaders used for home pedicures). Often our feet are so crammed in shoes we can't get our toes to move and spread during exercises. This helps stretch out your toes and helps you learn how to engage these muscles.

Consider stretching classes

- **Yoga.** If you're careful not to over stretch, yoga's perfect, but too much flexibility makes you unstable and can create overuse injuries in aerobic activities. Yoga is a great barefoot activity to help strengthen your feet.

- **Dance.** While preparing for my coast-to-coast skate, I took introductory ballet classes. Although I was constantly humbled by my 5-year-old cohorts, the classes were fantastic for strengthening the feet, core, and stabilizing muscle groups. Choose whichever dance class interests you the most, but make sure you can do it barefoot, or in a minimalist shoe. One dance method to try is modern dance, which is essentially done barefoot. Note, if you try ballet, look for the widest slippers you can get your hands on and feet in.

- **Eric Franklin Method.** This methodology was originally designed to help strengthen and improve dancers' form while reducing or eliminating injuries. Since barefoot running is essentially dancing while you run, there's incredible carryover between the Franklin Method and barefoot running. These classes can help strengthen and condition your feet as well as help you learn proper form and alignment.

- **Body Rolling.** With inflated balls, 5 inches in diameter, you can roll yourself out and elongate the entire muscle. This technique gets deeper into the muscle. Both Yamuna and RunBare have these inflatable balls available.

- **Martial Arts and Tai Chi.** There's a reason martial artists go barefoot or wear minimalist shoes that let their feet and toes feel the ground. Getting grounded, centered, and balanced by feeling the ground is essential for nearly every martial art. As you practice a martial art, you'll be developing foot strength and coordination, as well as core strength, and coordination between your feet and the rest of your body.

Rolling Stretches

One of the biggest challenges I often face with the traditional medical community is their approach of looking at any "one" problem in a vacuum. This approach often treats the symptom, rather than the cause. That's particularly important when we're talking about the feet since every part of your body is connected. You're like the marionette mentioned earlier, with connective strings pulling to hold and move you. Relaxing one part, results in moving another. We're a giant chain or system of ropes and pulleys—each of which pulls on the feet.

So far this chapter has discussed foot conditioning and strengthening, but foot conditioning extends beyond the feet. Not only do we have 19 muscles of the feet, but we have 13 muscles and tendons that connect our feet to our legs, then legs to our pelvis, and so on.

If you've been stretching like crazy, and your feet are getting tight, or you feel as if you can't overcome internal resistance in your feet, it may not be your feet at all. Another part of your body may be pulling on your feet. The key is to work on balancing and symmetrically strengthening your body. Grab a foam roll and tennis ball or RunBare or Yamuna ball and make sure you're stretching out all parts of your legs, plus your hip flexors, psoas, and glutes.

Recently, the top of my right foot became sore. Despite constantly stretching and backing off further, the soreness wouldn't go away. Turns out, the problem wasn't my foot at all. It was my hips becoming imbalanced again because I was not staying active enough while writing this book. As the hips become imbalanced, the right hip is forced to do more of the work. This pulls on my back, pulls on my glutes, pulls on my quads, my calves, and then on my feet.

Like with me, your feet are your weak link (or have the smallest muscles, tendons, and ligaments) and are where you'll likely feel the "problem," even though it may not be a foot problem at all. Once I identified the weakness, I began stretching out my hips more, and almost everything else along my legs. Suddenly, the tightness in my foot went away. Here are some exercises to help you smooth out some weaknesses:

- **Rolling Over a Ball (and seeing it spread out).** Earlier I mentioned using a golf ball for strengthening exercises, but golf balls and other similar balls (such as the RunBare foot ball) can also be used for stretching too. Rolling your feet over a golf ball or other hard ball is a great foot massage that helps loosen up your muscles and tendons. With the golf ball under foot, slowly roll the ball around the bottom of the foot while seated or standing lightly. If you find any tight spots, keep the ball there for a few seconds to a minute, then move along slowly. Make sure you start into this slowly, or you may bruise or strain the bottom of your foot. However, over time this exercise will help keep your plantar fascia loose, as well as give additional flexibility between your metatarsals.

- **Squashing Chicken Feet.** Standing with your foot flat on the ground, picture your foot as an imaginary triangle, with the front of your foot as the base (like that of a chicken) spreading between your widest contact points on your forefoot as you squash and flatten your foot. Flatten, then release and repeat for a count of 10.

- **Rolling Arches.** Standing with your foot firmly on the ground, roll your arch inside toward the ground as you gently squish your foot down to the inside, and roll your foot back up to the outside. Squash and roll side to side, for a repeat of 10 times.

- **Pull Back.** This is similar to a very basic hamstring stretch, except we're focused on the foot. Sitting on a mat or on the ground with your legs extended out in front of you, gently pull back on one forefoot (do not go to the point of pain) and hold for 10–20 seconds, then repeat. Repeat at least 3 times.

- **Log Roll.** Sitting in a chair with your foot out in front of you, hold your foot with your opposing hand, with your fingers on top of the forefoot, and your thumb under the ball of your foot. Picturing your foot or metatarsals as a series of logs, gently roll the logs (and your foot) as you roll the logs back and forth. Hold in each direction for a count of 3, then repeat in the opposing direction. Move slowly and repeat for a count of 10.

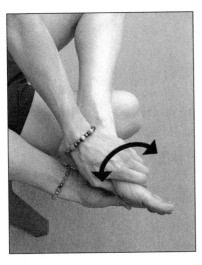 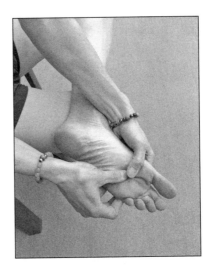

Log Roll: Gently roll your foot to the outside, and then back in, imagining your metatarsals as logs, rolling back and forth as you gently roll out your foot.

- **On Your Knees.** Kneel on the floor with your feet straight behind you, gradually work on lowering yourself back without bouncing; this will stretch both your feet and your quads, though our focus for now is on your feet.

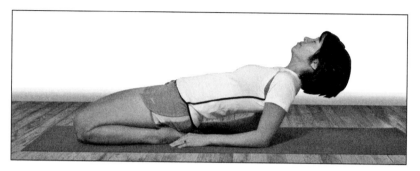

On Your Knees: Work to bend back exceptionally slowly. Do not bounce or force it. You aren't trying to rip your quads in half, just gently stretch out your feet. Never do this stretch with cold muscles.

For each of these exercises, I recommend beginning with a set of 10. After a week or two, progress to 2 sets of 10, and finally, 3 sets of 10. Work on going slowly with proper form, rather than rushing through these. It's best to teach your muscles to move individually and correctly, rather than using brute force and muscling them all at once.

In all foot movement, you're shooting for gaining mobility, flexibility, strength, and control. You don't need to do all of these in one shot. Mix it up as often as you can to give your body as much variety as possible. Whatever you do, take your time, and have fun with these!

The Foot Externals

I've often talked about feet having eyes—in other words, the sole has the ability to sense the terrain and maintain balance. It's said our soles have a "dynamometric map" for balance and control. By feeling the ground, they greatly assist in keeping us upright. In short, the feet act as an incredible biofeedback mechanism, sending valuable information to our nervous system to help control the incredibly sophisticated task of staying balanced.

In essence, "The feet at the ball and the heel act as two antennae that repeatedly scan the ground," according to *The Human Foot*, a textbook written for podiatric school students.

Feet were meant to feel the ground. They're not just equipped with more nerve endings than almost anywhere else on the body, but with more *types* of nerve endings.

There are 4 different kinds of mechanical receptors or mechanosensors in the sole of the foot, including sensors for vertical pressure, local pressure, skin stretch, and rapid tissue movements.

If you've ever stepped on a very sharp object or came down hard on a rock, you also triggered nerve endings or pain sensors that respond to high levels of force and pressure. Other types of nerve endings respond to lesser, dull pain in already damaged or inflamed tissue, such as when you've formed a blister from repeated stress to the foot. Both of these sensors work together to keep you out of harm's way from acute injury or overuse.

Unfortunately, when you place your feet in shoes, you deaden or eliminate the effectiveness of your entire sensory feedback system.

To me, dogs are exceptional barefoot runners. They have the most incredible pads on their feet and, with proper conditioning, can run just about anywhere and everywhere. They've got thick skin on their pads, little grippers to keep them from sliding, and amazing fat deposits underneath, exactly the qualities barefoot runners strive to obtain.

Not to worry, our feet aren't going to look like Fido's. In fact, great bare feet don't look ugly at all. Sure, they look a bit more natural, but since they're not squeezed into a shoe, they don't develop bumpy bunions, calluses, or corns. The skin looks thicker, both on the bottoms and the sides (to protect the sides of the feet from rocks and give you more stability).

Build Pads Just Like Your Dog's Feet

Our feet are more like our hands than we think, helping us grab and hold onto things. We have specialized pads on the ridges of each of our toes and across the soles of our feet that help keep us from slipping and sliding across uneven or slick surfaces, and for running at speed. These pads have additional sensory receptors along the ridges of our skin. And they have a unique second feature: sweat ducts that work together with the sensory receptors to give us additional grip with our feet.

In short, our feet were designed to help us grab the ground and maintain traction. (Unlike rubber, our feet were designed to gain traction once they get wet.) This is yet another feature or benefit designed by nature, yet eliminated by shoes.

We often think of fat in our bodies as bad or unhealthy. But not when it comes to the feet. Our feet have vital subcutaneous (under the skin) fat pads, which are essential for protection of the foot and for shock absorption.

When I talk about building pads, I'm referring to developing the thickened skin and fat deposits underneath. When you start into barefoot running, most likely the skin on your foot may be baby soft. There's an important benefit to starting with soft skin. Soft skin helps keep you from over working your muscles, tendons, and ligaments when you begin. Over time you'll notice two changes:

1. The skin on your feet will grow thicker and tougher.

2. More fat deposits will accumulate beneath the skin on the bottoms of your feet.

I've inspected a lot of feet since I've gotten into this game, and I've discovered several stages we transition through as we grow our own shoes. Now, some people are born with thicker skin or more padding than others, but we can all grow thicker padded feet.

Stages of Pad Development

1. Soft and tender skin gets compacted (moisture is squished or packed out) and begins to thicken for natural puncture protection.

2. Fat begins to get deposited under skin to act as natural shock absorbers.

3. Skin begins to harden to protect against blisters.

4. Skin begins to get shiny and "plasticized," particularly if running on man-made surfaces.

5. As layer after layer of skin is deposited, foot becomes thicker, even to the sides. Over time, you can expect a few millimeters up to a centimeter of growth. (Yes, you DO literally grow taller!)

6. Extra cushioning continues to be deposited to your thickened skin.

7. Gains become permanent—meaning, the padding you've grown will last even through the winter.

◉°°°₀ FOOT NOTE

How do you make thick skin? Your plantar skin (skin on the bottom of your feet) is naturally 600 percent stronger than skin elsewhere on your body and can grow even thicker—up to a centimeter—but only if you use it. As you start to go barefoot, you wake up this potential for "skin of steel" on your feet. Running barefoot both stimulates additional skin growth on your feet (layering) and pushes the moisture out of the skin (strengthening). Together, by adding layers of skin, and by strengthening the skin, you thicken the soles of your feet.

Grow your own armor

During the adjustment period, you can expect to experience scuffs and small cuts. As long as you're not rushing things, though, these will be minor nuisances rather than serious injuries. And whenever your skin heals from such nicks and tears, it will grow back stronger.

It will take months until you have "living shoes" that are both highly sensitive and able to shrug off collisions with unexpected objects. Once you toughen up, though, you'll be surprised at what your feet can tolerate. I've found I can stand and run on broken glass with no harm.

One important caveat is to beware of substances that reduce the hardiness of your feet. For example, if you run on water or snow, it will soften your pads. That's okay if you remain on such mild surfaces for the remainder of your run. But if you switch to a rougher surface while your feet are tender, they're likely to become raw and injured.

The same goes for running in shoes—even minimalist shoes—that make your feet sweat (and so tender), and then taking the shoes off in the middle of the run. Always consider the state of your feet when selecting what ground to run on and always run barefoot first, then put on the shoes—never the reverse.

As long as you maintain continual awareness of both your running surface and your body, your "living shoes" will make the chances of a serious injury relatively small.

The bottoms of your feet have more sensory receptors than almost anywhere else on your body. When you're in shoes, you can see these receptors at work because you develop calluses, or thickened, hardened skin, wherever you have an irritation with the shoe. What happens is the sensory receptor sends a message to the brain saying there's an irritation, and the brain sends a signal back to the foot to grow the skin thicker at the area of irritation. Calluses then grow, which are nature's way of protecting your feet.

We use this same feedback mechanism to grow thicker pads on our feet for barefoot running. When you first run barefoot, you stress the bottom of your feet. This sends signals to your brain to lay down more skin to protect the feet. As new layers of skin are laid down and as you continue to run, you push the moisture out of this skin. The thicker your skin, the more protection you have, and the less moisture in your skin, the stronger it is and less susceptible to wearing down or being punctured.

To grow this thicker skin, you must work the skin (run barefoot) and then rest the skin. If you don't give at least a day or two between barefoot workouts, you'll just keep wearing down the new skin you're trying to build. Expect your skin to feel hot and tender after your early workouts. This is your body's way to both stimulate growth and throw additional blood flow to your feet to grow additional skin. Respect this heat and the growth by resting between these workouts. It'll be a few months before you're ready to run daily on your bare feet, but if you give the skin the time it needs, you'll be there before you know it.

Sure-fire ways to stimulate pad growth

Want to grow pads fast? While you can't rush Mother Nature, here are some elements to consider exposing your feet to. Just remember, your skin grows slowly for a reason. It's to keep you from doing too much. But with that said, the following list may help with your pads.

1. **Pressure.** The more pressure you put on your skin the better. Now this doesn't necessarily mean going out with a backpack full of bricks. This does mean that running will stimulate pad growth faster than walking, since you land with more pressure or downward force when you run. Just take this in stride, until your ligaments, tendons, and bones can handle the pressure. Resist the urge to go fast.

   Pressure and pain. If you step on something that makes you wince, as long as you're not bleeding on the spot, rest assured you're doing your feet some good. Those small pressure points will heal to grow stronger, thicker, and faster. (Unfortunately, it's often the outsides of your big toes that take the biggest hits from pebbles. Ouch! This does help the feet, but can hurt like a bugger!)

2. **Duration of Contact.** Over time, the more distance you put on your feet, the better. Time on the feet is essential, and barefoot walking is much better than nothing when it comes to pad development. Just be sure not to go too far and scuff your feet raw. Build up slowly and rest in between.

3. **Intensity.** The faster you go, the more pressure you put on your feet. Not only does this mean running will generate pads faster than walking, but it means that running up hills where you're really pushing into the ground to lift yourself up the hill can be a great way to develop pads without extreme effort. Even walking uphill on the balls of your feet is a way to grow your own shoes quickly.

4. **Dirt and Trails.** I recommend all road runners spend time in the dirt for their feet. When you run on the roads, only your contact points with the roads get stronger and tougher. The skin under your arches stays far too soft. This can be dangerous for stepping on sharp objects or rocks on the path.

   Not only do dirt surfaces provide natural pressure spots (small rocks and other things) to stimulate quick growth, but the dirt seems to aid thickening of the skin. Dirt and trails have the added benefit of positively affecting and protecting more of the foot. Even if you're a pure road runner, this can come in very handy. (While this isn't directly pad related, dirt and rocky trails have the added benefit of making your foot muscles stronger, suppler, and more flexible, which all help prevent overuse injuries. Additionally, it increases blood flow for recovery and flexibility for protection for the entire foot.)

The only time I truly cut the bottom of my foot, I'd been running on the roads for weeks. One day nature called as I was running and I jumped off a paved path and into the woods for a quick relief. Unfortunately, I landed straight on a broken stick with the soft part of my foot. It skinned my arch good. Had I been running more on dirt, I would have had more protection.

5. **Heat.** Our bodies are amazingly adaptable, if we start slowly enough. To me, nothing beats heat for quick skin and pad development. The hot pavement also feels good underfoot, once you're used to it. But you must start slow, or dance with the heat in extreme moderation.

   Moderate heat or even excessive heat can stimulate skin growth fast. In springtime or your first runs in heat, pay careful attention to pain, and let it be your guide. Avoid blisters or burns by stopping early and putting on your shoes. By the time your feet feel toasty, you're already doing damage.

6. **Cold.** While heat is my favorite, I love the cold too. Why? Because our bodies are amazing at adaptation, and cold is another great stimulator of foot changes and growth. Moderate cold, not done until frostbite, can greatly increase pad development and vasculature to the foot. In a later chapter I delve deeper into how to prepare for barefoot running in extreme temperatures.

7. **Sand Sprints.** Is there a playground or volleyball court or beach near you with fairly coarse sand? If so, and it's clean, use this sandbox for building your feet. Walk, jog, or if your feet can handle it, even consider a half dozen or so short sprints in the sand every other day or so. A sandbox is ideal for conditioning and strengthening all of your skin on your feet, even in between your toes. It's a great exercise for strengthening the skin and, if you do sprints, for strengthening your entire foot. Again, just build up slowly, and let your skin be your guide.

Surprising pad building shortcuts

Apply the tips in this section only if you have been barefoot running for a minimum of 3 months or more. Letting your pads be your guide is critical to your success as a barefoot runner. If not, you risk overuse injury or permanently taking yourself out of the game.

Other than time and Mother Nature, there are no perfect solutions to pad building. At best, it can be said that good form, time, and recovery are your best solutions. Many of these solutions I've borrowed from climbers, martial artists, gymnasts, baseball players, and even musicians keen on plucking strings.

At present, building strong pads is an imperfect science. I hope in the future we'll have more scientific studies to help determine what stimulates pad growth the most.

- **Sand.** In the book *Indian Running* (a book on the lore of Native American running, the majority of which was once done barefoot), one runner was said to have filled his sandals with sand, presumably coarse, to help keep his feet conditioned over the winter. This might work on soft ground or snow, as long as your feet stay dry and the sand doesn't turn to clay or mud. It does have the added advantage of getting all parts of your foot. Just be careful it doesn't change your stride, particularly when running on the rough stuff.

- **Sandpaper or Emery Boards.** Many climbers scuff up their fingers to help skin grow back stronger (and they also do this on problem spots to prevent the skin from cracking). I haven't tried this yet, though I have deliberately scuffed the soft parts of my feet on my cement stairs at home to stimulate and strengthen soft skin. Just be careful not to scuff too much. Start slowly and see how your skin reacts.

- **Chalk.** Rubbing your feet with chalk can help keep your feet dry if you're in shoes, or to condition your skin after a run. I find this works well at keeping the skin dry, without causing it to crack in dry conditions. You can find chalk balls at your local climbing store or gym supply store. Personally, I prefer the eco-friendly Metolius Eco ball found at REI stores.

- **Tannic Acid or Strong Tea.** Tannic acid is a chemical found in oak leaves you can find at many natural pharmacies. According to a 2002 article in *Podiatry Today*, soaking the feet in strong tea or a tannic acid solution (consider a 10 percent solution) may help toughen the skin of the feet.

- **Rubbing Alcohol.** From climbers to lifters and more, I've heard that wiping your skin (in this case, feet) at least twice daily with rubbing alcohol helps dry out and toughen your skin. I've tried this extensively, but unfortunately, in the dry climate of Colorado it doesn't seem to work. Instead, in dry climates it promotes dry and cracking skin. However, it may work in more humid climates or after your feet get wet. One possible combination solution: dry your skin with alcohol, then oil the dried skin once or twice daily to prevent cracks from occurring.

- **Salt Solutions.** Soaking in a salt solution may have a similar effect to rubbing alcohol. Many climbers swear by it to dry out and toughen the skin. Again in Colorado, this doesn't really work, but it makes me think of surfers and people who live near the beach. The skin on their feet grows incredibly strong, perhaps because of a combination of salt and sand.

- **Tincture of Benzoin.** This has been recommended by climbers and even runners for years for preventing blisters and toughening the skin. Tincture of benzoin is a strong-smelling benzoin resin from alcohol. It's recommended that you paint it on your feet or soft skin once or twice daily. Personally, I tried this for a few weeks, and though it was helping, I found it to be a mess and quite aesthetically displeasing. My feet turned varying shades of yellow and, despite proper hygiene, appeared dirty. Since I've worked so hard to take care of my feet, this solution didn't seem worth it. However, some Native American barefoot runners have sworn by tincture of benzoin or similar products for nearly a century.

- **N-butyl-based Cyanoacrylate.** A long name for the active ingredient in a product such as QuikCallus, which is touted as a medically safe version of SuperGlue for wound care, blister prevention, and protecting fingers and calluses. While I haven't found it to directly accelerate callus growth, it has allowed me to go out at times I'd otherwise be grounded. However, I don't want to use it on soft and weakened skin that needs time and rest to recover. Instead, I've used this as a preventive measure. If I know I have to run on rock-salt covered roads, wet chip and seal, or another surface that could hurt my pads fast, I've been tempted to give this a go. The result? It usually protects the skin for a few miles. I just have to be careful, because if I'm over-protective of the skin, I'm likely to hurt what's on the inside. This is not a great daily solution, but there may be a time and place for it.

Here's another possible use. If there's one or two areas of your foot, such as your big toe, that keep getting scuffed up while the rest of your foot is doing fine, or if you have a nick or scratch that's almost fully healed, but still sore to the touch, a little dab may help. Here you can use such a product to protect the worn or healing skin (never use on an open wound), but be careful and watch your form. It's entirely possible your stride is off, which is causing the skin to wear down your skin in the first place. If so, these products will only help promote poor stride and may enhance your chance of injury.

A better solution may be a new product called Goober Grease or products for climbers such as Climb On!, which helps heal cracks and worn skin.

Note: Many climbers and musicians swear by SuperGlue, in particular to repair thick skin that's been skinned or damaged (musicians call it "instant calluses"). Personally, I admit to having used it and find it dries faster and is stronger than QuikCallus. However, I CANNOT recommend it because it's NOT recommended by doctors as safe (it's considered an irritant) and may harm the skin over the long run. It was used by emergency doctors and nurses on the Vietnam battlefield to close wounds. There is now a medical-grade version of SuperGlue called 2-octyl-cyanoacrylate, which is used by LiquiBand, SurgiSeal, and others.

- **Pickle Juice.** I've heard soaking your feet in pickle juice can prevent blisters and help grow thick skin fast. Baseball Hall of Fame pitcher Nolan Ryan is said to have soaked his hands in pickle juice to protect his skin from his 100 mph fast balls. Gymnasts and weightlifters are said to have soaked in pickle juice to thicken the skin on their hands too and to prevent rips, tears, and injuries. It sounds interesting and perhaps worth a try, albeit pickles have a strong smell. One suggestion: finish your jar of dills and use the juice as a soak.

- **Urine.** Common Web lore has it that gymnastics coaches and weightlifting coaches recommend this for their athletes. Supposedly midstream urine is an antiseptic and helps cleanse and condition the skin. One technique is to use it while in the shower. I've heard of runners using urine to both condition the skin and help heal cracks from dry skin. I've even read from ESPN that sluggers, specifically Moises Alou and Jorge Posada, use urine to toughen up their hands for hitting. It seems to have been a common practice in ancient times too. I am passing on this idea, but my recommendation is that you stick with your own urine!

The trick with all of these methods is that pad building is a biological response to stress and pressure, in particular. All of the previous suggestions promote drying of the skin, but none help with compacting or packing down of the skin. To build good pads, you really need both.

Top 7 Ways to Maintain Pads during Inclement Weather

1. **Run Whenever Possible.** Run on dry pavement or dirt any chance you get as long as your feet aren't too cold. Dirt's preferred over pavement, but

take whatever you can get. Run at a good pace, but not too fast, and warm up your feet first.

If there's a chance of salt on the ground, make sure to wash your feet afterward and use oil to protect the skin and keep it from cracking.

2. **Head for Your Mall.** Do you have a mall with stone tiled floors? People are often found walking or jogging in malls during early morning hours. Consider walking or jogging barefoot at your mall once or twice a week. While it's always best to wash feet after workouts, make sure to wash your feet after the mall. These floors are NOT as clean as nature.

3. **Make Friends with a Treadmill.** While treadmills can change your stride (more on this in the chapter on maintenance) and overall aren't the best, they're far better than nothing when it comes to maintaining your pads. Start slowly, vary the incline, and work those pads. Just don't go too far or too fast, particularly in the beginning, or you'll run your feet raw, blister, or both.

4. **Protect Your Pads.** If you run in snow and water, make sure you don't soften your feet then hit coarse dry pavement. Instead of protecting your pads, you'll end up scuffing skin off. These conditions don't promote pad growth, but if you love running these conditions, consider using products such as QuikCallus to protect what pad you have left.

5. **Feel the Ground.** When you can't go barefoot, use shoes with an ultra-thin sole to feel the ground. This helps maintain and stimulate fat padding growth just beneath the skin.

6. **Keep Your Feet Dry.** If you're stuck in shoes or in boots, make sure you keep your feet dry. This helps you hold onto the skin you've worked so hard to get. Consider chalking your feet before and after each time you put them in a shoe. And make sure your shoes can breathe and keep your feet dry.

7. **Beware of Rock Salt.** Rock salt is incredibly sharp and dangerous for bare feet. The only time I got cut on glass was after rock salt tenderized my feet like a roast. Salt is literally a meat tenderizer, and rock salt can quickly turn toughened skin to mush. It's insidious too because it can hide in melted snow or runoff long after visible crystals disappear. Running in this water then softens your feet, turning harmless little pebbles and debris into dangerous hazards. Over time, rock salt leads to severe skin cracking, particularly in the spring.

The effect of duration and speed on pads

When it comes to pads, both duration and intensity wear your pads down fast.

- **Duration.** Run farther and you'll wear down your pads more. This is true both on challenging terrain, such as a rocky trail, and on very smooth paths, where you don't watch your form and start scuffing your feet (keep that core engaged, stay tall, and make sure your feet are going in the direction of travel).

- **Speed.** When beginning barefoot running, you don't want much intensity because your muscles, ligaments, tendons, and even bones need to adapt. Your skin tells the tale underneath. If your skin's fatigued, chances are everything else needs to recover as well. Adding intensity for pad growth before your feet are ready may tear up everything on the inside, leaving you injured and unable to run for months.

Even with good form and stronger muscles, pads wear faster when you pick up the pace. For instance, a seasoned barefoot runner may be able to run a half-marathon or more at a decent jogging pace. But if that same runner goes all out, a 5K at full race pace may be all she can handle. Speed wears padding faster than miles. So which is better for building pads: duration or speed? A mixture of both is recommended, but only after your first few months.

Pampering Your Feet for Recovery

With all of these exercises, and with barefoot running in general, your feet may get sore and tired. This is normal, so as long as you start slowly and never work out again until your feet feel fresh and recovered, you'll do great. You can take these additional steps to aid with recovery.

- **Ice Down.** In the beginning your feet may get noticeably sore after a workout, run, or strengthening exercise. I recommend cooling your feet off after workouts with 5 to 10 minutes of icing, and repeating 2 or 3 times if necessary. Personally, I like the Mueller Cold/Hot Wraps. They're inexpensive, infinitely reusable, and allow you to Velcro the icepack to your foot. It's clean, easy, and fast. I always keep a few packs ready in the freezer.

- **Elevate.** If you've had a really good workout and your feet or legs are wobbly, prop them up on a chair or wall to let your feet and legs drain. This leaves your feet feeling lighter after your workout and gives you a chance to rest, relax, and breathe as well.

- **Foot Massage.** You never need an excuse for a good foot massage, but if you've been working your feet hard, I especially recommend you get one. Foot massages help loosen the muscles, aid with flexibility, relax tense muscles, and aid with circulation—in other words, it doesn't just feel great, but helps your feet to recover and grow back stronger. You can have one professionally done by someone at a local massage therapy school, by a spouse, or even do a self-massage on the foot (see *Self-Massage for Athletes* by Rich Poley and Tim Benko or *Reflexology Massage* by Monika Schaefer for more on this). If you have the bucks, you could even buy a mechanical massager at Brookstone or other electronic gadget stores. (Consider a unit with a strong vibrating motor such as the old Acuvibe in which you simply place your feet on the machine. The strong vibrations efficiently increase circulation and loosen up your feet.)

- **Foot Rollers.** These help work out the knots in your feet like a golf ball while aiding in recovery and blood flow. Just work into this like golf ball exercises lightly, letting "feeling good" be your guide. Here we're concentrating on recovery, not on over-working the foot.

How not to pamper yourself

- **Pedicures.** I admit I'm not an expert when it comes to this luxury. But a common pedicure experience is to exfoliate or remove dead skin on your feet. In essence, they sand all your hard work away. I'd recommend avoiding this.

- **Hot Tubs.** Until gains become permanent, pads wear down too fast if your feet are wet. This isn't just about watching where you run, though running or hiking on coarse or cold surfaces with wet feet may scrub off your hard-earned skin. But it's particularly something to watch for if you're a triathlete, swimmer, or love to spend time in a hot tub. We've all seen our skin look like prunes after we're out of the water. Even a long shower or bath can temporarily soften our skin. Make sure you don't go barefoot running until your feet are completely dry and your skin is once again firm to the touch. (Early on, I made this mistake once. After a swim at the gym I stayed in the hot tub to loosen up and stretch. Then I headed home and out for a run. Though I'd been regularly running 5 to 10 miles a day barefoot, within half a mile I was raw and bleeding. My soaked skin had gotten soft, and I instantly wore off my hard-earned gains.)

Getting to Know Your Feet

I used to think my feet were ugly, though I never gave them more than a second glance. But that was *before* I began going barefoot. Now I check out my feet, and the feet of those I'm coaching as well. It's exciting to see people's feet change and adapt, almost before your eyes. Checking your feet out daily and after your runs helps prevent injuries and keeps your skin in great shape. Our feet can tell us a lot, if we take the time to listen.

Inspect your feet before each run. Is the skin still soft and tender? Are there any cracks to watch for? Any nicks or scratches you may not have noticed or areas of concern? Any tweaks of pain you hadn't noticed? And are they ready to run again? By watching your feet, you'll learn about your body; figure out what's right and what's not, what's working and what could be improved.

Self-knowledge and awareness are the keys to barefoot running and perhaps to life as well. The better you know your feet, the happier you'll be. Happy, healthy feet are the name of the game. Take care of your feet, and you'll go far.

12-Week Plan to Barefoot Running

Where to begin: I recommend starting on the smoothest surface you can find. As Steven Sashen, founder of www.invisibleshoe.com puts it, "Smooth surfaces give you the most information [sensory feedback]." This information is important to find a great stride and to grow your strong feet.

Your path toward stronger feet:

Smooth Paths → Choppier Paths → Easy Trails → More Difficult Trails → Gravel and Sharp Rocks → Speed

Gradually, start working into more challenging terrain. Perhaps go from smooth cement or a paved bike path to another manmade trail that's a bit more choppy and uneven. From there, as your feet grow stronger, begin to venture out onto dirt trails, perhaps with walks before runs.

Next, venture onto rockier surfaces such as chip and seal roads, and more challenging trails. If the trails are especially challenging, start out sans shoes, then put them on for your return. Never be afraid to put the shoes back on once your pads are toasted. Last, make peace with gravel roads. If you can get these down, your feet are good for almost anything.

Note: The following weekly plan is a general guideline and will vary from individual to individual. Everyone's skin adapts at different rates, irrespective of how good a runner you are. You have to go slow, and let your skin be your guide.

Step 1—Growing New Skin

When:	Weeks 1–2
How Often:	Every 2 to 3 days
What:	Easy Jogging
Where:	Smooth Cement or Paved Paths Only
Distance:	A Few Hundred Yards to 1 mile
Objective:	Stimulates Feet to Grow New Skin

Begin on the smoothest surface you can find, with very short distances to begin (perhaps a few hundred yards to start). Run until your skin feels a bit toasty, warm, or raw and not until you start bleeding. Instead, your feet will begin to feel tender. At that point, put on your shoes and go home. Tender is your stopping sign.

To grow your skin, rest between workouts. This is no different than the well-known rule of resistance training: Give at least 48 hours for muscles to heal from weightlifting. You never want to run on your tenderized skin. This prevents growth and creates blisters. Instead, let the skin grow back for a day or two, then head out again.

For up to 24 hours after a workout, expect your feet to feel hot. This is a good thing. You've increased blood flow to your feet. Your brain's increasing circulation to your feet to grow them back stronger and lay down new skin.

Step 2—Stimulating Padding Growth

When:	Weeks 3–4
How Often:	Every 2 to 3 days
What:	Jogging
Where:	Slightly Rougher Asphalt
Distance:	1–2 miles
Objective:	Stimulates Feet to Grow Padding

After a few weeks, you'll likely be up to a mile or more purely barefoot. It's now time to begin heading out on slightly rougher terrain.

As new skin is laid down, your feet begin to feel stronger. You can still feel small pebbles underfoot, but nothing's quite as fragile as it was just a few days or weeks before. At this point, your body begins to deposit more fat to the bottoms of your feet. You can stimulate this process by running a bit farther, or venturing off the smooth path and onto ever-so-slightly more challenging terrain, such as a paved path that's not quite buttery-smooth.

More challenging terrain and repeated stress sends further signals to your brain, which begins to lay down fat deposits for cushioning. Thicker skin develops, followed by thicker cushioning.

Additionally, you are stimulating the bottoms of your feet by stepping on small rocks or pebbles. Even the ones you don't really feel are sending signals to the brain to produce more cushioning; in essence, the tough stuff underfoot triggers the body's response to deposit more natural cushioning to that area.

Step 3—Hardening Your Skin

When:	Weeks 5–8
How Often:	Jogging every 2 to 3 days; Hiking once per week
What:	Jogging and Hiking
Where:	Jogging on chewed-up asphalt; Hiking on trails
Distance:	Jogging 2–4 miles; Hiking 1–2 miles
Objective:	Harden and strengthen your skin

After a month, you can begin to increase your distance to a few miles or more. Now is when the greatest changes begin to occur. Your skin goes from thin but strong to something far denser.

To harden the skin, it's now time to begin venturing onto tougher terrain. At this point I recommend occasional hikes, perhaps once or twice a week, on a fairly challenging trail. I'd keep it to a mile or two. Work on staying on your toes (to build the muscles you'll need for running) and prepare to slip back into shoes. These short hikes help "temper" the feet, or make them stronger than iron.

Step 4—Shiny, Happy Feet

When:	Weeks 9–12
How Often:	Jogging every 2 to 3 days
	Hiking once or twice per week
What:	Jogging and Hiking (Feel free to slightly increase jogging pace on smooth surfaces)
Where:	Jogging on trails or chip and seal roads; Hiking on trails
Distance:	Jogging 3–5 miles; Hiking 1–2 miles
Objective:	Strengthen skin to a whole new level, greatly increase foot strength and flexibility

If you've come this far, give yourself a pat on the back, now you're in for really fun stuff! After the first few months, the skin begins to radically change. Not only does it become denser, but smoother and almost plastic-like, particularly if you spend much time on manmade terrain or in the heat.

Now you're almost ready for daily barefoot runs. For the time being, pick up the pace a bit, while concentrating on proper form and more challenging terrain. Also, begin to add intensity to your runs, such as running uphill. Remember, distance and speed are inversely proportional. If you increase speed, you must decrease duration, and vice versa. Pads wear down through distance or speed. So if you pick up the pace, cut back on the distance. Venture out farther, perhaps 3 to 4 miles or more, and experiment with loose rocky terrain or chip and seal roads. Just check your ego at the door and continue to bring your shoes along.

For quicker pad development, remember to keep your runs every other day. This is important for the internals of the feet as much as for the externals. Additionally: alternate workouts. If you run fast for one workout, go slow the next. If you tried trails one day, head for a silky-smooth path the next. Alternate the terrain, surfaces, inclines, and more. The more you can expose your feet to at this time, the better, just stay moderately slow, let your skin be your guide, and resist the urge to run two days in a row. If you can't resist, head out for a barefoot WALK on your days off.

Consider alternating surfaces too; there's nothing better for building your feet than hopping back and forth between a rough trail and a smooth path. Hit the trail until the skin fatigues, hop back on the smooth path, recover, then repeat.

From weeks 9 to 12 you'll see maximum gains, in terms of your padding, foot strength, and flexibility.

Step 5—Pads of Steel (Week 12 and Beyond)

It's now time to play. Your feet will continue to grow, thicken, harden, and grow stronger, but you've passed a critical point. Your feet can now handle occasional back-to-back runs, along with a bit of speed. Just watch for your form if you go fast. Poor form can scuff up your feet and scrape off your skin. So be the tortoise and step into speed, slowly.

You can now venture out onto almost any surface to play. Gravel roads and sharp rocky trails may still be a bit away, but they'll come over time. Remember, your feet have had a lifetime in shoes; it will take many more months, if not a few years, before your feet fully adapt. The majority of African runners who compete so well on the international scene spent the better part of their first 18 years growing up, running, and racing barefoot. It'll take time to grow your full feet of steel, so give it time.

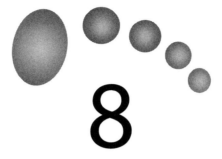

8

Barefoot Runner Maintenance Tips and Tools

If you run, you are a runner. It doesn't matter how fast or how far. It doesn't matter if today is your first day or if you've been running for twenty years. There is no test to pass, no license to earn, no membership card to get. You just run.

—John Bingham

The human body can handle almost any challenge or stress if it gets accustomed to it gradually enough. That's why karate experts can chop through cinder blocks with their bare hands and why great barefoot runners can leap from rock to rock and run for many miles over extreme surfaces. But they didn't develop such skills overnight—and you shouldn't try to either.

This applies even if you're already an accomplished athlete. That's because your body adapts to very specific activities. For instance, if you're a great marathon runner but you've spent your whole life in shoes, the skin of your feet will still need to gradually toughen. And if you've been heel striking in shoes for your entire life, you'll need to slowly get used to landing on the balls of your feet.

You also know there's a lot more you can do to improve your health and stride than mere running alone. To become the healthiest you can be requires work on alignment, flexibility, strength, rest, and proper nutrition.

In this chapter we'll look at fun ways to help you achieve your health goals. We'll get you fitter in the off-season, look at ways to make you stronger year-around, and help you with that all-important recovery. We'll do drills, balance work, strength training, stretching and more, helping you get started on the right bare foot.

In a nutshell, the process is as follows (think of building your feet in terms of weightlifting and building new muscle, which is exactly what it is):

Step 1. Overwork your feet very slightly. A small percentage of muscle fibers in your feet are torn down.

Step 2. Stop and rest, providing your feet time to recover. Your miraculously adaptable body responds by growing the muscle fibers back stronger than before.

Step 3. Repeat Steps 1–2. Very slowly but surely, your feet grow stronger and stronger.

As you continue this process—gradually and patiently, over the course of several months—you're likely to develop marvelously strong feet that let you run bare for long periods, and even under extreme conditions, without significant harm.

While it may seem counterintuitive, this process of going "slowly" is actually the fastest—as well as the safest—way to develop your feet.

One of the things to keep in mind while building up your feet is the 10% Rule. It states you should never exceed more than a 10% gain in activity (a total of duration, distance, and intensity) in a given week.

For example, if you ran for 20 minutes one week, then you can run 22 minutes the next. Or if you ran 10 miles one week, you can run 11 miles the next. Or if you ran 5 miles per hour one week, you can run 5.5 miles per hour the next.

Of course, 10 percent is a rule-of-thumb guideline. For example, if you haven't exercised at all for a while, change it to a 5% Rule.

The point is to set an appropriate limit and not go beyond it. Otherwise, you risk a cumulative overuse injury. You might not feel pain right way, but mounting damage can sneak up and bite you with a severe tear or break down the line. That's what happens when many people—bare or shod—go for an easy run and, seemingly out of nowhere, experience their feet or legs giving out. Nothing special happened during that particular run; it was just the last straw in a series of abuses over the course of weeks that finally pushed tendons, muscles, or bones past the breaking point.

The Dangerously Wrong Way to Condition

Unfortunately, runners hearing such slogans as "No pain, no gain" and "What doesn't kill you makes you stronger" often misinterpret them to mean that it's a good idea to push themselves relentlessly without carefully listening to what their bodies are telling them. They may even read popular books that immortalize runners who have "broken through the barriers" and "pushed past the pain."

As a result, they'll overwork their feet, and then overwork them some more, without providing adequate periods for rest and recovery.

In other words, instead of tearing down muscle fibers and then giving them a chance to grow back stronger, they tear down fibers and then tear them even more, providing no chance for healing and rebuilding. Since the damage is cumulative, even if they don't feel pain right away, they're injuring themselves further and further as the days and weeks go by.

Eventually, the results of this abuse are tears in a foot's tendons, muscles, or even fractures in the bones themselves. This leads to pain and inflammation that can take many months to heal. So their attempts to rush through a transition to running bare actually have the opposite effect by preventing them from running at all.

Going from broke

When I got into barefoot running, I was a broken runner. Overuse injuries, imbalances, and more had brought me almost literally to my knees, which weren't all that healthy either. Turns out, that wasn't a bad thing at all. It forced me to build back slowly while allowing my body to recover. It liberated me to experiment too; with nowhere to go but up, I could try to find the best ways to heal and grow back stronger.

At a recent clinic, I advised a struggling runner with plantar fasciitis to recover, then build back slowly. His response, "That sounds great, but I need to train for my next marathon." How many of us have said something like this? Unfortunately, your body doesn't know it needs to race again, it knows it needs rest. If you don't give it the rest it needs, you'll never recover.

Many runners struggle year after year limping along. Until you're ready to let go of the goal, to build back stronger, a cycle of pain continues. Sooner or later, you need to step back, take a break, and start from scratch.

Becoming the best runner you can be isn't about brute force, discipline, or training harder. It's about training smarter, by being aware, feeling the ground, and feeling your body. Instead of training on intellect, you're training with intuition. This may sound ambiguous, but the biggest challenge for runners has never been a lack of work ethic or the ability to push oneself; instead, it's been an inability to go slow, go with the flow, and listen to one's body. It requires a degree of mental flexibility that's hard when you have goals. However, when you force anything, something has to give, and something always breaks. I don't want that to be you.

My best advice: Don't do everything at once. Rather, pick and choose what seems like the most fun and go for it. Try new things out and feel free to mix up the routine. Our bodies are incredible at adapting to new challenges. So don't get stuck in a rut. Instead, change things up as much as you can. This helps work muscle groups you never knew you had and loosen you up in ways you once thought impossible, so you can become a balanced athlete.

Barefoot Drills

Drills actively help you gain strength, coordination, flexibility, and balance. Done properly, they can be a cornerstone to your success. You can choose from an infinite number of variations. Just focus on proper body position or form as described in the earlier chapter on getting started. Stay on your toes and keep your pelvis neutral in all exercises. Keep your belly snapped to your spine, your chest wide, and that silvery string pulling you toward the sky.

Remember, you're training your mind as much as your body—in essence rewiring your mind with each step. When you make a movement, you connect two neurons in your brain and each movement becomes a new physical connection. Over time, the neural connections become more permanent, and the movements more fluid. The trick is, if you perform the exercises in a sloppy fashion (such as bending forward or landing flat-footed), you'll wire sloppy connections. Focus on proper form over quantity. Less is more. Hardwire good moves and stop if you start getting sloppy.

Where to begin

Consider practicing these drills on a soccer field, baseball field, tennis court, or track with painted lines. Once you get the hang of things, work on quick, fluid, yet snappy motions. Before you're done, you should feel as if you've been doing a dance.

Incorporate the following drills into or before your runs two to three times a week. Consider doing drills such as Eagle, Goalpost, Rewind, and Shuffle during the middle of your runs, as well. Part of the goal is to keep you flexible, strong, and balanced by doing different movements. So if you feel like hopping, skipping, or running sideways during your run, then go for it. The more you work your feet and legs in different ways, the healthier, more economical, injury-resistant, and stronger barefoot runner you'll be.

Core drills

These drills focus on strengthening core muscles.

Eagle Wings

Purpose:	Builds core, arms, and shoulder strength, balance, coordination, and efficiency
Do This:	Lightly jog and extend your arms straight out to your sides at shoulder height. Continue for approximately 50 feet. The goal is to concentrate on a tight core and keeping your upper body from bouncing. Make sure you're not letting your head wag from side to side.

Over time, consider incorporating a few minutes of the Eagle into your regular runs.

Imagine This: Visualize your arms out to the sides like the wings of an eagle or a plane.

Goalpost

Purpose: Builds core, upper back and neck, balance, coordination, and efficiency. This is a great drill to keep your head from bobbing around while you run.

Do This: This is a slightly more advanced version of Eagle Wings, except run with your arms out straight above you. For best results, practice both Eagle Wings and Goalpost.

Imagine This: Visualize your arms raised above you like football goalposts.

Turnover drills

The following drills promote a high stride cadence.

Hot Feet

Purpose: Leg speed and fast feet

Do This: Run with the smallest, shortest strides you can take. Don't be concerned with getting your feet high off the ground. Stay on your toes, but keep your stride length to a mere few inches.

Imagine This: You're running on hot coals and you can only keep your feet on the ground for milliseconds at a time.

Showtime

Purpose: Works on getting your leg up for faster leg turnover by coordinating your psoas, glutes, and core

Do This: Bring your knee up to 90 degrees or higher. Hop on each foot twice, then switch feet. As you hop, lift your opposing leg as high off of the ground as you can, by driving your knee toward the sky.

Imagine This: Visualize a string pulling each knee toward the sky.

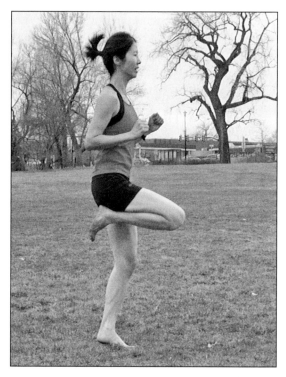

Butt Kick: Don't kick behind you. Instead, work on kicking straight up underneath you, bringing your upper leg to horizontal.

Butt Kick

Purpose:	Helps bring your leg around quickly
Do This:	As you bring your leg beneath you midstride (not behind you), kick up your foot toward your butt. If you can make contact with your butt, great!
Imagine This:	Your foot and leg are working together like the piston on a steam locomotive wheel (or like riding an exaggerated unicycle).

Bounding drills

These drills help muscles and tendons become more elastic and snappy for quicker speed, agility, lightness, and recovery. They also strengthen fast-twitch muscles, helping you sprint, avoid obstacles, and fly on downhills. In addition, consider making up your own drill for this one, a hopping drill on the fly, bounding from step to step, or footfall to footfall.

Bunny Hops

Purpose:	Works on building springy feet and legs by strengthening your ankles, Achilles, and calf muscles
Do This:	Keeping your chicken wings up, with both legs together, hop forward

about a foot. We're not looking for big air here. Hop on your fore-foot, but stay low to the ground. These should not be giant leaps, but small, fast, bunny hops.

Imagine This: Should look like a bunny hop line dance

Skip to My Lou

Purpose: Helps turn your legs into springs, while working on leg speed and quick steps

Do This: Keeping your feet low to the ground, hop on each foot twice, then switch feet.

Imagine This: Picture a child skipping, or that you've just gotten a job promotion.

The Rewind

Purpose: Keeps opposing muscles strong and helps prevent injuries by working on stabilizing muscles. This exercise also helps strengthen your feet, Achilles, and calves by encouraging you to stay on your toes.

Do This: You must stay on your toes to go backward with any grace. Run backward for 50 feet. Concentrate on staying relaxed and fully upright. Do not bend forward at the waist. This is another drill you can practice at length during your runs, particularly if your legs need a break to recover. Simply turn around and run backwards a bit. Just make sure you look behind you on occasion for safety, alternating looks from one side to the other.

Imagine This: Backing away from a mama bear and her cub

Lateral drills

Lateral drills are particularly important for injury prevention. They help strengthen your stabilizing muscles, giving you the anchor and stability you need to move without excess motion, wobbling, or the chance of an overuse injury particularly on trails.

Do the Shuffle

Purpose: Helps build hip and knee strength, improve joint function and stability, and protect your IT bands from overuse

Do This: With your arms out to your sides like the wings of a plane or a giant cross, move your left leg to the left, then bring your right leg to meet your left leg, then repeat. After 50 feet, switch directions so that your right leg leads and your left leg follows.

Imagine This: Pretend you are moving side to side with a giant racquet on a tennis court waiting for your opponent's serve.

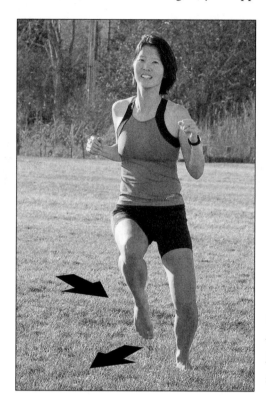

Gorillaz: Jump forward to the side (at a 45-degree angle) for each stride, bounding first left, and then right. Keep your upper body tall.

Gorrillaz

Purpose: Builds strength, stability, and helps you stay centered

Do This: Step forward (almost a controlled jump) 2 feet forward and 2 feet to the side (in other words, your leg should move forward at a 45-degree angle). As you land, stride forward with your other leg, again 2 feet forward and 2 feet to the side from your body (or 4 feet to the side from where your other leg landed). This should look almost like a forward moving pendulum below your waist. Your upper body should stay centered (over an imaginary center line).

Imagine This: Visualize running through tires while keeping your upper body centered.

Side-to-Side Crisscross

Purpose: Gaining coordination and learning to keep your weight centered as you strengthen your external obliques (side abdominal muscles)

Do This:	Run directly to your side for 50 feet while crisscrossing your legs with each step. Going first to your left, cross your right leg over your left leg. Then, bring your left leg out from behind your right. Repeat for 50 feet, then return in reverse, now crossing your left leg over your right leg.
Imagine This:	Picture yourself dancing like Gene Kelly in *Singin' in the Rain*.

Run the Line

Purpose:	Helps maximize efficiency by teaching you to keep your legs directly beneath you while strengthening your core and preventing excess movement
Do This:	Standing tall with your core engaged, run along a painted line directly beneath your feet making sure each foot lands squarely on the line directly in front of the next (on the grass or on a path). Make sure you keep your arms pointed forward, so they're not crisscrossing your body. This should be a very light, finesse-oriented exercise, with a tight core and your feet close to your body.
Imagine This:	Visualize running on a balance beam.

Forward Crisscross

Purpose:	An advanced version of Run the Line, this exercise promotes an efficient stride by keeping your legs incredibly close together. We're also teaching you to keep your feet straight, especially if you have a tendency to walk or run with your feet pointed outward.
Do This:	Keep your core tight and arms pointed forward while running with one foot crossing the other while running on a painted or imaginary line. Cross your right leg over your left leg and vice versa with your left leg always landing to the right of the line, and your right leg always landing to the left of the line.
Imagine This:	Walking on a curb, and each leg over-exaggerates each step (the left goes a bit too far to the right)

Twist 'N Shout

Purpose:	I learned a version of this one on a run with Erwan Le Corre, founder of MovNat. Helps build lateral core and lower back strength.
Do This:	This is a toughie! While keeping your legs moving forward, rotate your upper body to the right for 4 steps, then to the left for 4 steps.

Repeat. (For an even more advanced modification of this drill: still moving forward, bring your legs slightly to the left while your upper body faces right. Go for 4 steps, then reverse.)

Imagine This: You're turning your head to check out the cute guy or gal you've just run past, but instead of just turning your head, you're turning your entire upper body while maintaining your forward direction. Watch out for those pesky telephone poles.

Barefoot Games

Native American kick-stick and kick-ball races

Until the 1940s, Native American tribes had a rich tradition of relay racing and running games, typically centered around 4-member teams kicking a ball or a stick. No one knows for certain why they disappeared in the U.S., but they were an essential part of Indian culture. From the time children could run, they'd be found kicking a stick or a ball. In fact, many wouldn't run without the stick, and it's said to get people in from the fields quickly, they'd throw a stick down before them and then sprint.

These games helped produce stronger runners, many of whom went on to become long-distance messengers. These feet were capable of kicking a 3-inch stick for hour after hour, from 20-mile races covered in 2 hours, to overnight games encompassing the better part of 100 miles or more.

In Christopher McDougall's book *Born to Run*, he talks about the game of kick ball played by the Tarahumara who would kick a ball through the Mexican canyons while running straight through the night.

Many other tribes, such as the Pimas, Papago, Maricopa, and Yuman, also played kick-ball races, while many more tribes played kick-stick racing. The Zuni (kicking a blessed 3-inch tik-wa or kick stick) are the best known for their epic kick races, but it was also played by the Hopi, Taos, Navajo, and many more.

Kick-ball and kick-stick races weren't merely solemn games or prayers, but a way to communicate and compete with other tribes. These races were also a favored source of entertainment. From the time kids could run until they were in their 50s, they'd play kicking games, and even when they could no longer play, they would wager on the teams.

While kick racing is for the most part gone, it can be as useful today as it was back then in building strong feet, balance, stamina, and coordination. Stories and pictures depict people playing kick stick barefoot through cactus-riddled prairie lands at modern racing speeds for hours on end. If we can get our feet in even half the condition of these famed kick racers, we'll have some of the strongest feet around.

I can see many benefits from this fascinating game.

- **Stronger toes, both in terms of strength and of skin.** Kicking the stick will scuff up the tops of the toes, particularly important for hiking and running trails with branches or large rocks where you'll occasionally smack or scuff a toe. You'll also scuff up the skin between your toes as you grab for the stick. This soft area rarely gets use until you accidentally get a branch or rock jabbed between them on the trails. This game helps protect these surfaces against such unexpected dangers.

- **Building foot strength.** To juggle, grab, or kick the stick you'll strengthen your feet in ways, angles, and dimensions just not possible with traditional running. This additional strength, particularly by your small and stabilizing muscle groups, will help your feet become better balanced, making you less injury prone and stronger at whatever you do.

- **Greater flexibility.** Since you'll have to move your feet in ways they're not used to, not to mention under and over a stick, or placing it between your toes, your feet will naturally become more flexible, aiding further with future injury prevention.

Hot potato

Work on passing a golf ball from your foot to your partner's foot as fast as possible. Turn this game into a competition to see which team can pass around the ball first.

Follow the leader

Running around a park or along a bike path, the leader alternates from drill to drill with all members following suit and mimicking. A variation of this would be to have the leader do one drill, then pull off and go to the back while the next leader does a different drill, followed by the next person and then the next, until each person has had a chance to lead with his or her own individual drill.

Building Core Strength

Every movement in barefoot running should be anchored with the core. Running from the core keeps you light on your feet, and from doing unnatural, harmful motions like overextending your stride, and keeps you centered for optimal power and speed.

To become a great barefoot runner, you must work on core strength, stability, and balance, balance, and more balance.

Balance exercises

Want to reach up and get something, then you need balance. Stepping out of a car onto ice? Again you need balance. Want to be strong in all of your motions and activities while preventing a possible injury? Well, you've got it, balance is the key. Balance will help you in life, and in everything you do.

So how do you get balanced for barefoot running? First, start walking on your toes more, with your core engaged and a string pulling you toward the sky. This helps you condition your feet and legs and improves your alignment throughout daily activities. You can do this at the mall, the grocery store, walking to work, or even at home. Walking on your toes helps work your stabilizer muscles and gives you better balance for all of your activities.

Second, work on balance exercises either on a flat surface or using a teeter board, inflatable disk, inflatable half ball, or even a balance ball. I recommend beginning the following exercises while standing on the floor or ground for a few weeks before graduating to an inflatable disk or half balance ball. Once you graduate to the inflatable device, start with both feet on the disk or platform of the half balance ball. After 2 to 3 weeks, work on doing each exercise with one leg at a time on the ball. The more exercises you do with one leg at a time, the better balanced, stronger, and injury resistant you'll be. While I recommend a set of 8 to 10 repetitions to begin, if the going gets tough, trust your gut and cut the workout short, or reduce the number of repetitions. Over time, work up to 3 sets of 8 to 10 repetitions or more.

These exercises are some of the best (and therefore most difficult) exercises for strengthening your core and directly translating your balance to barefoot running. In the beginning, allow 2 days between each workout. If your legs or feet get sore, ice-down after your workout, and never do this workout 2 days in a row. Maximum benefits will begin after your first 2 to 3 weeks and occur if you're doing these exercises at least twice a week.

The goal for these exercises is to gain single-leg coordination, strength, and balance, while learning to engage and use your core for each movement. This will help with barefoot running efficiency, balance, injury prevention, and speed.

For each of these exercises, snap your belly button to your spine and snap your core together (both belly and spine) as tightly as you can with each movement. Begin with an exhalation while bringing the core in tighter, followed by an exhalation in the reverse.

Jumping Jacks

Start by standing on the floor or balance board with your arms by your sides. Your weight should be centered over the balls of your feet, while you work on grabbing with your toes. Raise your arms up above you, as if you were doing a jumping jack, until your hands touch above you. However, do not jump. Do this to a count of 3, then return your arms back to your sides for a count of 3. Repeat for a set of 10.

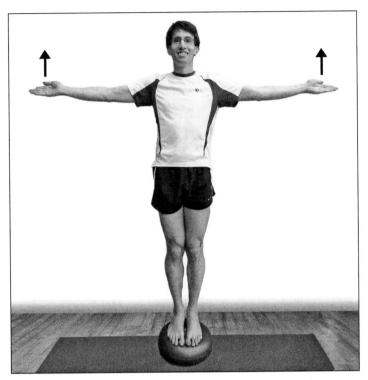

Perform Hundreds on a Ball by standing tall on a ball, teeterboard, or inflatable balance disk, with your arms to each side. Pulsate on an exhale with your hands facing down for a count of 5, turn the hands over and pulsate on an inhale for a count of 5. Then repeat. (For a more advanced method, stand with only one leg on the ball.)

Hundreds

While standing (or standing on a ball), bring your arms out to your sides, shoulder level, as if you were flying. Keeping your weight on your toes, pulsate your arms with the palms of your hands facing downward. Repeat for a set of 5, all within a single pulsing exhalation. Next, flip your hands so that your palms are now facing up. Now pulsate your arms for another set of 5, all within a single pulsing.

Knee Kick

With your arms out to the sides, bring your left knee up in front of you as high as you can to a count of 2. Return it to a count of 3. Bring your right knee up in front of you as high as you can to a count of 2. Return it to a count of 3.

Side Leg Raise

Same movement but with your leg out to your side, slow and controlled. Go as far as you can go, but with slow control.

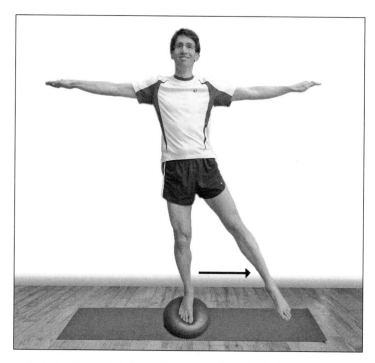

Side Leg Raise: With one leg centered on the ball or inflatable balance disk, bring one leg out slowly to the side, then back in and repeat for a set of 10. Then switch to the other leg and repeat. Make sure you stay tall and centered without leaning to the side.

Bow

This can be done two ways. The first is with your arms by your side. This is the less advanced method (lower resistance). The second is with your arms out to your sides. You can also do this standing on the ground, or as a more advanced method, on a teeter board, half balance ball, or balance disk (my favorite).

Standing with your feet no more than shoulder width apart and pointed forward, with your core tight, begin by leaning forward no more than 6 inches to begin. (As with the following exercises, this movement is about control, not about force or strength. It should be done with absolute control.)

Lean forward 6 inches, then bring yourself back to fully upright by engaging your core muscles and letting your core pull you back. There should be no arm or head movement, nor muscle movement from your pelvis, thighs, or butt. Simply tighten your abdominals and back and pull yourself erect. This should be a very slow exercise taking a full 2 to 3 seconds to move the 6 inches.

There should be no abrupt, sharp movements or throwing of your body. Repeat initially for a set of 10. Over time you can increase sets, range of motion, bring your arms to the side and, eventually, work onto a balance device. Again, focus 100 percent on control and movement through your core.

Back Bend

This is the exact reverse of the bow. Instead of bowing forward 6 inches, you're leaning backward 6 inches. Again you should pull yourself erect using only your core, or your abdominal and back muscles, nothing else. This should be a very slow and controlled movement, taking a full second or two to move 6 inches. (Repeat and increase difficulty as you progress.)

Side Bends

With your arms down by your sides, bend to one side to a count of 2, then reverse directions for a count of 2.

Pilates

Another great way to help hold your core in place is to do 10 minutes of Pilates exercises *before* you run. Pilates has a natural connection to barefoot running because barefoot running requires stability, balance, strength, and coordination that all come from the core.

Weight Training

I'm an advocate of natural training and natural running, so why do I advocate weight training?

I believe weightlifting can help you gain muscle strength and balance in ways that are initially difficult for beginner barefoot runners. Over time, as you work on balance ball exercises and spend time on the trails, you most likely won't need weightlifting anymore. Sure, you don't need it to begin with, but chances are you have some muscle imbalances. In other words, you may need to balance out muscles that are stronger, weaker, looser, or tighter than others. Personally, when I started into barefoot running I'd been weightlifting to recover from injury. This helped me make the transition quickly and effectively.

Weightlifting can help particularly as you get into a barefoot running program, or during the off-season (late fall through early spring in cold climates). Weightlifting helps with injury prevention, proper form, greater efficiency, and endurance, and for the performance minded, weight training helps with speed.

To get the most out of the gym, I recommend strength training 2 to 3 times a week. You don't need hard workouts here, just consistency. Work your muscles frequently, and they'll remember what you want and give you what you need.

The overload principle

As with all physical training, weight training works on the overload principle. Overload or strain the body slightly, yet repetitively, and as long as you give your muscles time to rest and recover, they'll grow back stronger. This is the same principle that kept our ancestors alive for millions of years. Chase after prey today and struggle? You'll get stronger for your next hunt. Barely get away from the saber-toothed tiger? That run too will make you faster for your next escape.

The overload principle works great, as long as you don't overdo it too much, too quickly, and as long as you give yourself plenty of time for recovery. Rest for at least one day before heading back to the weights.

In order for the overload principle to work, you must teach or train the body on a regular basis. In other words, one weightlifting session that gets you sore will do little to train and strengthen your muscles. You need to work muscles every few days in order for them to gain memory and strength. The first time you overwork something, it's unlikely the body builds back stronger. Instead, it just repairs the damage. But if done with frequency or repetition, such as 2 to 3 days a week, you'll become stronger, fitter, faster, and more resilient. However, if you don't give your muscles a chance to recover and grow back stronger, you'll just tear things apart instead of strengthening muscles.

Note: If you've been lifting for more than a few months, then any less than 2 to 3 strength training sessions a week may allow you to maintain your current strength, but won't help you gain strength. This may be fine during your peak running or racing months, but consider doing more during the off-season.

Muscle tone vs. muscle mass

When you're weight training in the gym, you're not aiming to gain "bulk." As barefoot runners, you don't need nor want to carry extra weight. Lugging around a huge amount of extra muscle won't benefit your muscles, joints, heart, lungs, or runs.

I'm also not advocating you become string-bean thin for barefoot running either. I've seen too many runners looking anorexic-thin. Even if that buys them another 5 to 10 seconds per mile, it's unhealthy in the long haul, causing undue wear-and-tear on the body. I want you to be healthy for a lifetime and not overly concerned about what the scale has to say, or what others have to say. To me, if you're happy, healthy, and running fast, that's all that matters.

Barefoot running naturally develops tone and strength, so it's unlikely you'll become a waifish-scarecrow while running barefoot. You may even shock yourself by how quickly you'll gain overall strength. When you run barefoot, you don't have an overbuilt shoe or cast on your foot to support your weight. All balance and support comes from your body. This extra "work" translates to a stronger pair of legs, core, and even upper body. You'll naturally gain upper-body strength, but without the bulk. You'll need a strong upper body as a counter balance to your legs. And it'll come naturally.

Michael's Rules for Strength Training

- **Train in Moderation.** Any extra weight you gain has to be carried by your feet and legs. Especially train your upper body in moderation.

- **Focus on Form, Not Speed.** Anyone can throw a weight, but that's not the goal. The goal is to lift the weight slowly with control. Lift with a 1 count, lower with a 2 count. Your maximum gains come on the down part of the lift, or the eccentric muscle contraction, so return the weight slowly with full control.

- **Build in Gradually.** Even if your legs are strong from barefoot running, the ligaments and tendons aren't ready for the new motions. They'll be foreign and create some strain for your joints in the beginning.

- **Listen to Your Body.** There's no set formula for how much weight to increase how quickly. Instead, just as in barefoot running, you must become more aware of your body and its needs.

- **Think Balance.** In every exercise you do, in each movement, seek balance between the right and the left, and each opposing muscle group. In other words, work out each leg separately. We all have a weak side and a strong side. But barefoot running is about a delicate, soft, balanced run. This means we need to correct imbalances in strength and stride equally with both sides.

- **Concentrate on Higher Repetitions.** If you're doing leg extensions, do a set of 10–12 repetitions with your right leg, then with your left. Remember to go slow and controlled.

- **Recover. Recover. Recover.** Always rest at least one day between weight-training sessions.

- **The 90-degree Bend Rule.** Stay safe in the gym by never exceeding 90-degree bends with your joints. If you're doing a hip sled, standing squat, or lunge, don't bring the weights so far down you bend your knees more than 90 degrees. The same goes for leg extensions or any other exercise. Always stop at 90 degrees.

- **Never Lock Your Knees.** The reverse is also true. When doing a hip sled or hamstring curl, never lock your knees or bring them fully vertical. Instead leave a slight bend in the knee so they're not forced backward or hyper-extended … ouch!

- **Stop Early.** Legs wobbly? Think you can do more? Stop. Save it for next time. Your goal here is slow steady building to help your barefoot running, not to risk injury while becoming the strongest guy or gal in the gym. It's too easy to rip, tear, or overuse muscles, especially when you're just working for a bit of tone, strength, and balance. Remember your priorities, and live to lift another day!

Weight-training plan for beginners

Run on fresh legs *before* you lift weights if possible. Barefoot running on tired legs not only promotes poor form but can lead to overuse injuries because your stride changes to accommodate your tired muscles, and your feet and legs aren't as elastic or flexible as you'd like them to be. Remember, running's the priority, not lifting.

For the first session in the gym, I recommend doing one set of each exercise, with zero resistance. For instance, if you're doing lunges, do a set of 10 to 12 repetitions without any weight. A set of hamstring curls? Keep the pin out, and again do one set of 10 to 12 repetitions with zero resistance.

Yes, for some it may seem ridiculously easy at first, but remember, you're not building muscle strength in the beginning, you're building ligament and tendon strength and the neural pathways to help the muscles learn the new movements and fire effectively.

At your second session (at least 2 days later), do 2 sets with zero resistance. If it isn't a struggle, move to 3 sets with zero resistance at your third session. After the third day of lifting (this should be after a week) begin by adding weight to your first set on the first day, 2 sets on your second, and 3 sets on your third. From there on out, the simplest rule is that if on your third set, you can comfortably do 10 to 12 repetitions at a given weight, increase weight for the next lifting session (for example, if you could lift 20 pounds for 3 sets on Wednesday, go to 25 pounds for 3 sets on Friday).

(Personally, I prefer lifting with a pyramid. So I would do one set at 15 pounds, 1 set at 20 pounds, then one set at 25 pounds. If that's too easy, the next time I would do one set at 20, one set at 25, and attempt one set at 30, and so on.)

I'd recommend being barefoot in the gym if it's safe and acceptable. This helps you feel the exercise better and work your toes, feet, and legs for greater balance. However, if it's not possible, acceptable, or comfortable for you, then no worries. An alternative is to use kung-fu or karate shoes (shoes for martial arts). These are basically slippers with a minimal amount of protection. They still let you use your toes to grab the ground and have free movement of your feet. However, they won't get you kicked out of the gym.

Being barefoot (or in minimalist footwear) in the gym helps you feel imbalances and asymmetries in terms of strength, flexibility, and form. Even upper body movements, such as bicep curls, are felt through the feet. Lift one side better than the other, you'll feel it. Jerking weight around instead of moving slowly with controlled movements, and you'll feel that too.

You could also try wearing many of the socklike minimalist shoes discussed in a later chapter, such as the Sockwa, Feelmax, or even the Vibram FiveFingers Mocs or Performas that have been specifically designed for indoor or gym use. The latter are much more like a glove than a shoe.

An argument can be made that you want more protection for your feet in case you drop a dumbbell or weight on your foot. However, if you have the misfortune of dropping a weight on your foot, unless you're in a steel-toed boot, any protection is likely too little. Best to be extra careful in the first place, never to rush, and be mindful of what you're doing in the moment.

Treadmills

Treadmills. Are they good or bad, and how do you get into them barefoot?

Approach treadmills with caution. They're a fantastic training tool but can bite you if you don't approach them carefully. They are, however, a useful real-world compromise for barefooting in the winter.

If you start slowly, the friction on the rubber does wonders for pad development. But proceed with extreme caution. A treadmill radically changes both stride and forces and can wear off your pads in an instant. Having a belt coming toward you, a control panel before you, and a cushioned platform all change your stride. Add a little ego to the mix, or desire to see your pace go up, and you can quickly get yourself in trouble.

To safely traverse the treadmill, follow 3 simple rules.

1. **Let the heat on your skin be your guide.** If your feet start getting hot, even if the skin looks good, call it a day. Never go to the point of blistering, and if you've scuffed your toes raw, give them plenty of time to rest.

2. **Never run the treadmill two days in a row.** In fact, if you're scuffing your skin up pretty good, don't use the treadmill more than every third day until the skin's grown stronger. Remember, if your skin's cooked, so is everything else on the inside.

3. **Never exceed your form.** If you find your form's getting sloppy, or you can't stay on your toes, slow down, back off, or go home. Running with poor form not only habitualizes poor form, but can get you hurt fast.

How to begin treadmill running

I recommend starting with 5 minutes, then adding a minute per workout. For the first 2 weeks, only walk on the treadmill. During the first week, keep the treadmill flat. During the second week, add a 1 to 3 percent grade. After 2 weeks you can try jogging, beginning at 3 to 3.5 miles an hour. Afterward, consider increasing your speed no more than a tenth of a mile per hour, per workout.

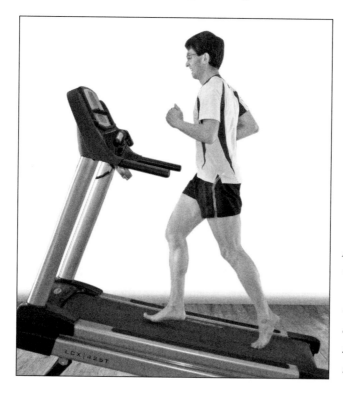

Treadmills, when approached with caution, can be a valuable tool. Warm up by walking or jogging on an incline at a slow pace to build strength and keep the impact low.

The goal is to increase distance, then speed, without sacrificing form. This gives ligaments, tendons, and bones a chance to grow stronger, without the risk of injury. I recommend beginning with a slight grade for warming up, then dropping it down as the going gets fast.

While adding a minute at a time may sound insignificant, it adds up quickly. Starting with 5 minutes and adding 1 minute per workout, you'll be at 20 minutes of light jogging within one month, 35 minutes in 2 months, and almost an hour of pain-free jogging within 4 months. Imagine running for an hour pain-free and fast! Done over the fall or winter, you'll transform into an amazing barefoot runner before spring ever begins. Best of all, you'll do it injury-free, while building form, strength, and balance for a lifetime.

As the saying goes, be the tortoise, not the hare. On the treadmill it's essential for your success.

Conditions to watch for

While you can work your way into your longest or fastest runs ever by using a tread-mill wisely, you need to be vigilant for signs of trouble such as changes in your stride, squeaky joints, strange aches and pains, or twinges of pain in your feet or your joints. Take note at the first signs of these trouble spots, and consider slowing down, shortening your workout, or taking a break.

You're more prone to overuse injuries on the treadmill because you're stuck on one flat surface that doesn't change, undulate, or vary. No rocks. No twigs and branches. No grass. No variation. With no respite it's easy to get into trouble. To avoid this, mix things up:

- Change the incline. Run a steep uphill for a minute, then flat, then some-where in the middle.

- At the same time, move forward on the treadmill, then back, then some-where in between.

- Vary your stride length, with some fast steps, and some a bit longer with-out overextending your legs.

- Vary your speed and even consider walking once every 5 to 10 minutes to let things cool down and recover (particularly for what's on the inside).

Running aware

When running a treadmill barefoot, you can't zone out or the treadmill may bite you. Temporarily shelve your MP3 or headphones and instead focus on form. You want to remain in a constant state of awareness, assessing your bounce, stride, fatigue, and signs of pain. If there's a TV screen attached to your treadmill, don't turn it on, but instead watch your reflection. Concentrate on your breath as you try to keep your reflection from bouncing up and down.

I like to repeat a mantra of thanks while making myself smile. Smiling helps release endorphins and healthy chemicals in my brain and throughout my body, helps keep me in a positive place, and keeps my ego at bay (particularly important because our ego always tries to make us run faster than we should on a treadmill or in any indoor workout where others may be watching).

Vibrams on treadmills

Many runners use the treadmill to work their way into Vibram FiveFingers or other minimalist shoes. There's nothing wrong with this, simply proceed with caution. As discussed in a later chapter on minimalist shoes, Vibrams and other minimalist foot-wear pose a unique challenge. They're more like bare feet, so they're incredible fun.

However, the muscles, ligaments, tendons, and even bones in your feet take time to wake up and aren't used to the new stride. Because you are not able to feel the ground, adjust your stride, and let your skin be your guide. It's too easy to do too much, too quickly.

On a treadmill, you may not even realize you have poor form until you've overdone it with your feet. Start barefoot, then incorporate minimalist footwear. If that's not an option, start extra slowly and watch your form (consider running by a mirror).

Cross Training for Barefoot Running

Cross training or doing activities other than running is a smart way to build form, strength, and fitness. By working on muscles you might not target with barefoot running, you build a better, more balanced athlete, prevent overuse injuries, become stronger overall, and keep your mind fresh.

So what do I recommend? There are almost an infinite number of possible activities you can use for cross training. If it gets your heart rate up, and works different muscles, then you're probably on the right track.

Cross Training Guidelines

When it comes to cross training, follow these key rules:

- **Do All Exercises 100 Percent Erect.** This means standing tall without leaning forward at all. Never stick your butt out, nor curve your back, but keep your core engaged, your back strong, and your posture tall. Remember that silvery string pulling you to the sky.

- **Let Go of the Rails or Hand-holds.** If you're on a stair-stepper or elliptical-type machine, don't hang on. Instead engage the core for balance and maintain your spring-loaded chicken wings (as long as it is safe, do not risk injury by doing something that may cause you to fall). This may be very difficult to do at first. If so, alternate one minute holding on, and then one minute with your chicken wings to your sides.

- **Stay Light on Your Toes.** At first this may be incredibly difficult for balance, so work on it slowly. The lighter you are on your toes, the more you're in a barefoot running position. However, depending on the machine, this may be very difficult to do at first and may require significant strengthening of your stabilizing muscles.

- **Watch Your Reflection.** Do the activity in front of a mirror if possible, and do your best to mimic your barefoot running form.

- **Have Fun!**

Cycling/Spinning

For myself, with my cycling background, I still love to go out once a week for a long bike ride, typically Saturdays. Then I tend to take Sundays off—a rest-day habit I picked up years ago from Japanese marathoners.

If you're injured and out of the running game for a while, as long as it doesn't aggravate your injury or a foot, get to know your bicycle. Your bicycle is one of the best cross-training tools you have. Just make sure to ride it barefoot … no, just kidding. But do ride, just like you run barefoot. Use a high cadence (leg speed) or fast turnover in a very low or light and easy gear. Feel free to go up all the hills you want, but remember to keep it in an easy gear and if things start to hurt, back off or head for home.

(If you're stuck indoors, either throw your bike on your trainer or rollers—devices that let you use your own bicycle as an exercycle indoors or right in your living room. Rollers (my favorite) allow you to ride and balance on your bike, just as if you're outdoors, working on balance in the process and helping you keep from going brain dead by forcing you to stay awake and keep steering and balancing your bike, or you'll fall.)

Take a spinning class for a fantastic workout and wonderful complement to barefoot running. I used to be a spinning addict in the winter. Perhaps it was because Wednesday evening classes, led by my Pilates instructor Don Spence, were a hoot! We'd have a regular crowd each week. Picture 12 of your closest friends stuffed into a small dark closet, strung with Christmas lights, the sound of techno music pounding out a beat, and a professional cyclist in the middle yelling, "You're stars, you're all stars … now ONE GEAR HARDER!"

Spin classes can keep you in shape in the winter, keep your leg turnover fast, and build great camaraderie. Take note, do not *lean* into the machine. Rather, engage your core to hold your body in place. I recommend if you're going to run on a treadmill the same day, do it before your sweaty spin workout. This'll help condition your pads and keep them in shape, rather than slough them off after your spin workout.

A safety note for spinning bikes and outdoor riding if you're recovering from injury. Out-of-the-saddle workouts are great, particularly when cross training, but when healing from an injury are likely too much on your body. If you're working too hard, healing, or if it hurts, don't feel bad about sitting down.

As a general rule for cycling, you might want to move your saddle farther forward—perhaps a few millimeters each week, to find a position that more readily duplicates your barefoot running position. In general, cyclists sit farther back than runners, so to simulate running on your toes, you need the saddle forward over the cranks or bottom bracket more. How far is too far? Gradually, go forward until you are bending your knees at more than a 90-degree angle, or until your foot is behind you at 90 degrees on the crank arm. Generally, it's unlikely your seat will let you go too far forward on a traditional bicycle, though it may be possible on a triathlon-specific bicycle where the seat tube is already more upright than a regular road bike.

Make only small saddle changes at a time, and as you come forward, you may need to raise your seat a bit. In general, the farther forward you are, the closer you are to the bottom bracket, and the more you need to raise your saddle. Make small incremental changes over weeks, if not months, so you don't aggravate your knees.

Swimming

To me, swimming's all about form, or learning how to relax and let the water carry you. Perhaps nowhere is the expression "go slow to go fast" more appropriate than in a pool, where if you try and go fast, you'll only fight the water and slow yourself down. Instead, you need to relax into your stroke, just as you relax into your stride, and then you'll get faster in the process.

Swimming is an all-around great activity that promotes a long, lean body, great upper-body strength, and fantastic core muscles (not to mention building stronger lungs and better rhythmic, diaphragmatic breathing). Furthermore, swimming with short fins on (such as Zoomers) for kicking helps and is a great workout. (It's also fun to fly across the pool with the fins on!) Alternating between swimming and kicking laps is an ideal way to help keep your legs toned. No, it's not the same thing as running, or aqua jogging, but it will get your heart rate up and help you if you're in the pool to heal from injury, and help you hold onto some of the muscle strength and tone you've worked so hard to get.

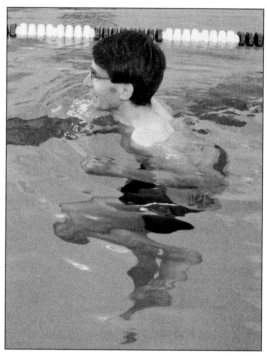

Aqua jogging is a great way to get in shape, tone neglected muscles, and hold onto fitness if you've been injured. All you need is a pool and a good flotation belt.

Swimming is tremendous for core strength, and for your back, and for working muscle groups you don't tend to target in barefoot running. Just make sure if you swim, your feet have dried for an hour or two before you go for a run. If not, your softened skin will slough away at the start of your run, leaving you in pain, and weeks or months from building back your pads.

A few years back a friend of mine, Yasuko Hashimoto, re-injured a knee from over-training just 6 months before her big chance to qualify for the World Championships in the marathon for Japan. Injured, her best chance to stay in shape was in a pool. She spent the next few months running up to 6 hours a day in a pool. She used an aquabelt to help her stay afloat and never touched the ground. It worked. She won the world-famous Nagoya Marathon to qualify for the World Championships in 2007.

There are several schools of thought around aqua jogging as to technique in the pool. What I tell my athletes is to try to use your legs to keep you as high as you can, while doing a pedaling type of motion. There's no real way to keep perfect form in the pool, but do work to keep everything pointed forward.

When you begin aqua jogging, you'll find water has far more resistance than you ever expected. So again, begin slowly, perhaps 10 minutes at first, then work up from there. At first, your small muscle groups, ligaments, and tendons, particularly around your knees, will be sore. They won't be used to moving or flopping all around and will take time to strengthen. But this is why swimming is so ideal for cross training, even when you're back up and running.

Stair climbing

When I was a teen getting into cycling, in the winters I used to head to downtown Boston and find the deepest underground subway station I could. There was one with an escalator so long it was often filmed for heaven scenes in movies (you can't see the top from the bottom). I'd head to this station late at night, when everyone was home, ready for the greatest workout of my life. I'd sprint the entire length of the escalator, up the staircase heading downward. Then I'd head back down and repeat. If I really wanted a workout, I'd sprint down the stairs as well, working on leg speed in the process.

What's so great about running stairs? Shod or unshod, you're on your toes. You'd have to try really hard to heel strike while running stairs. Any opportunity you can get, head for the stairs whether it's at home, in the stairwell of your local building, a baseball field, or a nearby sky scraper. Try it barefoot for one of the best workouts in the world (the best workout may be running steep trails).

To start, barefoot jog or walk 10 flights your first day (trying to stay on your toes). Rest for a day or two. Then add another couple of flights the next time you hit the staircase. You'll build calf strength without straining your Achilles too much. Just remember to stand tall and don't hinge forward at the waist.

Steppers, climbers, and other machines

Elliptical trainers and **StairMasters** are both excellent tools for maintaining aerobic fitness and muscle strength when you can't hit the trails or the roads. Again, work into them gradually until your joints are ready for the new motion. For myself, my shins start to get to me on the elliptical machines unless I build in slowly. It's quite unlike the motion of barefoot running. Your body may not be used to the motion of sliding backward and forward. Building into a stair stepper may be easier, but your knees and quads may not be ready for the workout, so start slowly there, too.

I recommend athletes do these either barefoot, or if they must wear shoes (most gyms frown upon unshod members) wear the most minimalist footwear you can get your hands on, such as a Feelmax shoe (more of a Kevlar lined slipper) or a Vibram FiveFingers such as their indoor Mocs or Performa.

Whether you're on an elliptical or a StairMaster, avoid holding onto handles and rails as much as possible. Instead, engage your core and stay light on your toes. This promotes proper balance and coordination between upper and lower body and helps you minimize upper-body moving and swaying, helping you become more efficient and less-prone to injury when you're back out barefooting. If your core isn't strong enough to hold you upright without holding on for long, then alternate between holding on and going hands free. Maintain the same form you would if you were barefoot running.

The **VersaClimber** is another exceptional tool. Stay on your toes, keep the resistance light, and climb for the stars. Try to use your upper body as little as you can (use the lowest hand-hold you've got in front of you), while keeping a high foot cadence. Be careful not to stick your butt out far behind you by keeping your pelvis level and standing tall.

Ski machines are awesome training tools too. When used properly, they help you stay on your toes. Just as with the ellipticals and steppers, try to stay light and let your lower body, not your upper body, do the work. Engage your core muscle groups and stay light on your toes.

I've heard that **rowing machines** are the life-blood of a true ultra-endurance runner. Personally, I've used this for cross training ever since I got into cycling. Rowers give you a total-body workout and, if done with high cadence, really help tone your back and arms. And for barefoot running, they're the perfect way to build shin, calf, and quad strength. They help you find your rhythm, develop strong breathing habits, and tone your upper body.

To start rowing, do 1 minute the first day, rest a day, then 2 minutes, followed by 3. I never build more than a minute a day so I don't burn out the ligaments and tendons in my arms. I like rotating my arm position, a minute with the hands facing down on the grips, a minute facing up. This works different upper-body muscle groups and keeps you better balanced. Pull in to your chest, not to your waist. Remember not to use your back to pull, but your core muscles and keep the resistance light. Finally, it's much better to work at a high cadence with lighter resistance (just as you run) rather than pull on the machine with all of your might.

While training for my cross-country skate, I had a discussion with Lisa Smith-

Batchen, one of the most winning triathletes and ultra-endurance athletes in the world. I was struggling back then with shin and foot pain, and she had some excellent advice for strengthening my lower legs—spend time with a jumping rope and a rowing machine.

As simple as it is, **jumping rope** is one of the best cross-training activities out there, particularly for barefoot runners. Why? Because it gets you on your toes. That's one reason that many people with debilitating knee pain can still jump rope—because they're no longer heel striking.

Since it's an explosive jumping exercise, start slowly both in terms of duration (how long you jump) and intensity (how fast you go and how high you jump).

Other Activities

Tennis, soccer, racquetball, and any sport that has you running around on your feet can help you cross train. I don't recommend them for injury recovery, but I do for working on lateral stability. Playing a game of tennis or soccer a few times a week helps strengthen ankles and joint stability. If the court's not too coarse, or if you're playing racquetball indoors, you may even be able to get away with going barefoot, and what a fantastic lateral-stability workout that is!

Always keep your core tight with these sports, never over stride and play in the most minimalist footwear you can get away with. In Latin America it's quite common for people to play soccer barefoot, and here you'll still see many Ultimate Frisbee players barefoot. Just judge the safety and camaraderie of the group in advance. If there's a chance of getting stepped on, or worse, SPIKED, keep some shoes on. (Note: I would not recommend playing sports such as Rugby barefoot, that really would make you a blood donor.)

There may be no better way to strengthen your feet than **barefoot climbing**. With the holds, varying terrain, and necessity to put all of your weight on a small part of your foot, it's ideal for building world-class pads and foot strength. But watch out. Unless you're ready for this, start with doing only one minute the first time, then build up excruciatingly slowly. Why? Because the same reasons it's an amazing foot strengthener are the same reasons it can easily be too much force for your feet. (If you don't start slowly, what an amazing way to build instant tendonitis!)

Don't jump off the rocks or a climbing wall thinking you can catch yourself with your bare feet. You'll get hurt. However, building into climbing slowly can be amazing for your new-and-improved monkey feet.

Barefoot running is just a small segment of all of the **natural movements** we did in nature since the beginning of human existence. Founded by Erwan Le Corre, MovNat (www.MovNat.com) helps you rediscover what it means to be human. You can build stronger feet for barefoot running and more. He founded MovNat to help people get healthier, stronger, and reconnect with nature.

Fitness classes, step classes, slide-board classes, Tae Bo, and just about all activity classes that do not have you throwing weights around are all cross-training opportunities. Just start into them slowly, listen to your body, and as much as possible do them barefoot.

Aerobic dance conditioning classes, in particular, are a fantastic way to get in shape and improve lower-body (and foot) strength and flexibility. Dancing simultaneously works on balance and core strength. Even if the class isn't very aerobic, there are still great benefits. As an ultra-endurance inline speed skater sponsored by Rollerblade, I signed up for ballet classes. Why? To improve balance, form, technique, core, leg, and foot strength.

Stretching

Want to stay healthy as you transition into barefoot running, pick up your pace, increase mileage, and just stay flexible and loose, in general? Want to work out all the knots and kinks in your muscles, all the tight spots, and imbalances?

For this, you need to stretch. Stretching helps you stay balanced and healthy. Additionally, it helps you get smooth and efficient. Ever wake up with creaky joints in the morning? If your muscles aren't loose, your joints are forced to do all the work. When you stretch, you allow your joints to move freely, rather than in stutter-step motions that pull and strain your entire body.

To get fluid, smooth, and ache-free, you need to stretch. I like what Dr. Nicholas Romanov, author of *Pose Method of Running* calls it. He says stretching is "oiling the body." You wouldn't drive a car without any oil in the engine, so why would you run without stretching out and allowing your joints to move freely?

Although new studies are showing that excessive flexibility has its drawbacks, tight muscles, or imbalanced tight muscles can be a serious challenge both for your barefoot running as well as your overall health. Tight muscles impede blood flow, wreak havoc with your form, and can cause serious overuse injuries.

When you're young and healthy, you feel invincible. But sooner or later this starts to change and you have to take care of things. And even if you're young, unless you've concentrated on bilateral exercises your entire life, one side of your body's likely tighter than the other.

If you're imbalanced, or have ever had an injury, then you'll likely need to stretch to get things even again.

There are many kinds of stretches and ways to stretch. When it comes to barefoot running, you don't need to become a master yogi. What you need is to become balanced, to prevent one hip or calf from being tighter than another. And you need to prevent and eliminate knots from your muscles. You need to focus on stretches that help bring blood flow to your muscles and eliminate knots.

Traditional stretching has its place, particularly if you've had an injury. For myself, with my titanium hip and femur, I need to keep up with traditional hip stretches. If not, my left leg, with the extra hardware, will become much tighter than my right and pull my entire body out of alignment.

As runners, we tend to hate doing anything that takes time away from our runs. However, time spent stretching will help you perform better and keep running for the long haul. It's basic maintenance that's an investment in your future. It'll add pleasure to your runs as you'll remain pain-free, while being more fluid, powerful, efficient, and fast. Time spent stretching is not time taken away from running, but a gift you give yourself to become a better runner for an entire lifetime—shod or unshod.

Stretch after every single run, after long travel in a car or on a plane, and especially on a day off or any time you need to rest. Rest days may be time off from running, but they're the best time to stretch, help the body recover, and allow it to relax and hit the reset button for a fantastic new week.

Dr. Romanov shares an inspiring story about Lance Armstrong. After the 1999 and 2000 Tour, Armstrong added an hour of stretching a day to his training routine. "The results were evident when he won the Tour of Switzerland and the Tour de France back-to-back in absolutely dominant fashion. Stretching not only improved his strength and power, but also helped him recover, a vital concern in stage racing. Over five weeks of intense racing at the highest level of the sport through June and July 2001, he never suffered a single bad day."

Types of stretches

As long as your muscles are warm, I find great benefits with both traditional and rolling stretches. Personally, there would have been no way to rehab my hip had I not spent a great deal of time working with traditional stretches to get my hip joint loose and mobile again. And it took heating things up, only by stretching in or near a hot tub that I was able to get the hip to relax and let its guard down enough for me to stretch and begin rehabilitation. A hot yoga class is another option.

Traditional stretches have been around for a long time. If done properly, they can be quite helpful, but all too often, people push beyond the point of pain, stretch when their muscles are cold, or overstretch, digging so deep they tear their muscles apart or loosen their joints. This isn't a real concern if these stretches are done in moderation and done when muscles are warm. These stretches are also best at stretching out the beginning and ends of muscles, but don't do very much to lengthen or stretch the belly or body of the muscle. For this we need to use a foam roll, ball, or other device to help dig in or knead out the muscle itself.

In these stretches you reach or extend as far as you can for a given period of time. Rest, then repeat. These stretches are progressive; therefore, you should go slightly farther each time you do them, yet never go to the point of pain or discomfort.

Traditional stretches can be done every day, but must only be done when you're warm. I recommend at least 30 seconds to a minute for each of these stretches. Ideally do a set of at least 3 of each stretch for maximum benefit. Also consider alternating between opposing muscle groups. For instance, work your quads and then your hamstrings.

Here's a great technique with opposing muscle groups. If you've been stretching your hamstring and it won't relax, try tightening your quadriceps for 10 to 20 seconds, and then restretch your hamstring. By tightening and then relaxing your opposing muscle group you help the muscles let down their guard (for instance, often the hamstring protects the quadriceps, and vice versa) allowing you to get a better stretch. Never go to the point of pain.

To perform rolling stretches, I recommend each of my clinic participants invest in a good foam roll and tennis ball (a stretching kit is available on our www.RunBare.com Web site). These tools are lifesavers.

Traditional stretches have their place, but often just work the beginning and end of the muscle, not the muscle bed or body of the muscle itself. That means the attachments are loose, but the body of the muscle remains tight and at risk of injury. Additionally, we often have trauma or sore spots within the muscle itself that feel like knots. These points of inflammation can develop into scar tissue over time, creating muscle imbalances and chronic pain. You can get at these knots and scar tissue with deep tissue massage and other techniques, but you can't get at them with traditional stretching. That's where the ball and foam roll come in.

You can use this technique for any muscle group on your legs, or even your arms (and I've heard of some people using it for their back as well, though I've never found much success with this). Simply lie down on the foam roll on the muscle group you want to work on. I tend to find great success with my athletes by having them lie on their side with the foam roll resting on their IT band, just a few inches above the knee. Then I'll have them roll down on the foam roll, inch by inch very slowly.

As they roll I want them to become aware of any tight spots, and if they find one (it's usually accompanied by pain), to stop on the tight spot, and just lean into it on the foam roll. Unlike traditional stretches where you don't want pain, here a little pain is a good thing. It's letting you know you've found a knot and are working it out. After a minute move on, seeking the next point of discomfort, tightness, or pain.

You can do this for your entire leg. As you start into barefoot running, a few key spots to work on will also be your calves and Achilles, and quadriceps. Work each of these areas out, doing the hamstrings as well, inner thighs, and even up to your psoas (group of muscles just before your groin that help you bring your leg forward as you run), which are often too tight, preventing a proper stride.

◐°°° FOOT NOTE

One of the best stretches I was ever taught was by Don Spence. In his Pilates classes, Don taught that many pulls, aches, and pains come from tight glutes where the IT bands attach to the hip. Loosening the glutes can literally loosen muscles all the way down to the feet, ankles, calves, knees, up to the hips, back, and more.

All you need for this stretch is a tennis ball and a grimace. Place the tennis ball on the ground and sit on it with one of your butt cheeks. Roll around slowly on the ball until you find your grimace, then live there for a minute or two. Roll on the ball for the first day for 5 minutes each side, and increase as necessary. You'll almost immediately feel muscle tension reduced in your legs and back.

Guidelines for stretching

Many of the basic prerunning stretches have been around for thousands of years. Stories of ancient runners, dating back to the time of the Romans, Greeks, and original Olympians, tell the tale of runners pulling, pushing, and contorting their muscles with bouncing motions just before the start of a race. These stretches may have actually hurt the runners, and definitely did little to help them.

Unfortunately, these same stretches are around to this day and likely have as little effect now as they did then. They don't work for two key reasons. First, bouncing or ballistic stretching as it's called, is a sure-fire way to hurt yourself if you don't build into it slowly and with proper form. Second, stretching cold muscles, particularly by pulling on them, tears fibers, rather than stretching them out.

Bouncing when stretching is a big no no. And cold muscle stretching is incredibly traumatic to the body. It should never be done, particularly by barefoot runners who rely so heavily on stability and balance from our muscles.

3 Best Times to Stretch

After a Warm-up. Stretch after you've been walking or running for at least 10 minutes. If you have a sore muscle, such as a tight calf or pulling hip, jog or walk for 10 minutes, then stop, and ever so gently stretch things out. This'll help you have a better run and keep you from injuring yourself or changing your stride due to tightness. You can even jog around the block, head for home, and roll yourself out on a foam roll before your run to increase blood flow and circulation to your muscles. This is particularly helpful if you have a hard workout coming up, such as speed work or a distance run.

After a Run. After you run, your muscles are nice and loose, as long as you haven't overdone things. Now is the time to work out the knots, keep things supple, and allow for the best possible recovery. Again, make sure you don't bounce, but with warm muscles you'll likely find you can easily stretch twice as far and with half the effort as stretching without a run. Stretching after a workout is one of the best things in the world you can do for recovery and to keep muscles from tightening up. Of course, if you've gone too far or too fast, stretching after a workout will only help so much. And if you're in pain or sense swelling, skip the stretch and head straight for the ice.

Once a Day. Stretch as part of a daily routine. Consider this as maintenance stretching, perhaps the most important kind. You can stretch any time of the day, although I recommend doing it at the same time each day. This helps you get into a rhythm or routine and ensures you get it done. Perhaps you do it after some core work in the morning, or after a Pilates class, or even in the evening when it's time to wind down. I recommend warming up the muscles for 5 to 10 minutes, and then going through a regular stretching routine, preferably emphasizing your foam roll and tennis ball. For instance, you could do a brief balance workout on the balance disk, then once you're warmed up, head for the (stretching) mat.

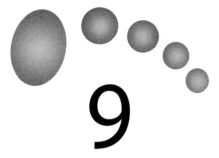

9

On the Right Track with Nutrition

Life expectancy would grow by leaps and bounds if green vegetables smelled as good as bacon.

—Doug Larson

Whether in a shoe or out, staying properly fueled is important for your runs, and when you're barefoot, it's even more important. Because when you're barefoot, you're going to be able to run farther, and likely faster, than ever before. You'll find yourself in new situations, new places, and with new abilities that demand proper fuel.

Perhaps you'll dare to run a 10K, marathon, or even an ultra. Or maybe you'll spend hours and hours trekking through the woods. Maybe you'll increase your mileage, or simply become a regular runner.

But to grow strong and healthy, to become the best barefoot runner you can be, or simply to succeed in participating, or winning whatever it is you do (using your own definition of success), you must be well fueled.

Although barefoot running is easier on your joints, it's a much harder workout than traditional running, at least in the beginning. Your body must adapt and grow stronger, from your muscles, to your tendons, ligaments, cartilage, bones, your core,

---

Michael Sandler is not a registered dietitian. Advice given here is gleaned from the athletic world's experts on sports nutrition and Michael's professional athletic experience. As with all medical advice, consult your doctor before making any changes in your diet.

your heart, and lungs. Everything must pick up the slack and do for you what your shoes once did.

In this chapter we'll look at what you need to know about nutrition to get you started on this journey and to keep you going and growing strong.

Eat More Naturally Every Day

The basics of eating more naturally aren't rocket science, just good ole common sense we've forgotten somewhere along the way. Here are the basic dozen principles for eating more naturally.

1. **Eat Organic.** Organic foods are grown a kinder gentler way, without potentially harmful chemicals, antibiotics, or genetic engineering. If our fruits, vegetables, and protein sources are getting bathed in chemicals, then sooner or later, these chemicals find their way into our bodies too.

2. **Simplify Your Vocabulary.** If you don't know what you're reading on the label, it isn't natural. Now that doesn't necessarily mean it's harmful. But if you can't pronounce it, or define it, you might want to keep it out of your body.

3. **Eat a Varied Diet.** This is just like saying run on varied terrain. The more varied our diets, and our runs, the better balanced we are, and the more we help our bodies. In simplest terms, you get different vitamins, minerals, and nutrients by eating fruits and vegetables of all different colors and tastes.

4. **Eat More Fruits and Vegetables.** If the colors and tastes of the rainbow are a natural pharmacy filled with amazing phytochemicals, vitamins, and nutrients, then wouldn't you want to eat more of this great stuff, and less of the empty stuff?

5. **Avoid Empty Calories.** Sugars, syrups, and fast-burning simple carbs do little good for your body. Think of maximum bang for your buck. If you're going for a run, you want the best trail you can find, right? So if you're eating, you want the best food you can put in you too.

6. **Go Complex.** The more complex your carbohydrates, or the slower they burn, the more nutrients they have and the better they are for your body. Grab a book or check online for the glycemic index of your favorite foods. Look for foods lower on the glycemic index to keep your mind and body happy and balanced throughout the day.

7. **Avoid Corn Syrup.** Processed and bleached sugars and corn syrup had no place in nature. Not only do they spike your blood sugar, they may be one of many reasons diabetes is at near-epidemic proportions today.

8. **Go Raw.** Think about this, ancient man didn't have a fireplace or any means to cook. Since we haven't evolved since then, likely neither have our stomachs. Ancient man survived for millions of years before ever cooking a meal; it's what our bodies adapted to. Try eating more fresh raw vegetables and fruits and protein sources deemed safe for a raw diet. Those who propose eating only raw say raw foods boost your immune system, increase your health and recovery, and give you incredible energy.

9. **Shun Preservatives.** Stay away from preservatives, additives, and artificial colors, flavors, and sweeteners. All those long names weren't found in your food in nature, so likely don't belong in your diet today.

10. **Go Simple.** The fewer ingredients the better.

11. **Go Local.** Local foods tend to be the freshest, best tasting, kindest on the environment (there's no fuel being burned to get the food to you). You also support your local economy. Look for a local food co-op to save you a bunch of money and get you the freshest, sweetest goods.

12. **Stay Away from Processed Foods.** You'll do much better with the fresh stuff and no added chemicals or sodium.

Staying healthy and at your best isn't just about the origin of your food, its chemicals, or the recipe. Things used to be simpler (and naïve). The biggest food choice was whether to use butter or margarine. Over the last few decades, food has taken on a controversy of its own: Fat was bad. But not all fat. Carbs were bad. Okay, some are not. Avoid too much protein. Trans fats, ugh.

To stay fueled and at our best, we need to understand more about our diets for peak physical and mental performance.

Carbs

When it came to running in the past, the general rule was carbs, carbs, and more carbs with minimal fat. But today, that's all changing. We're finding the body was never designed to eat such a high-carb diet. Additionally, carbs are rocket fuel; they burn quickly, raise blood sugar levels quickly, then crash leaving you feeling empty.

It turns out high-carb diets don't give you extra energy or prevent fat storage in the body, but can leave you feeling hungry, even when you're full, and tired and cranky once your blood sugar level crashes.

Fats

In nature humans ate more fat and protein. Healthy fats such as monounsaturated fats are actually healthy for our bodies. These include monounsaturated fats found in nuts, avocados, and olive oil, and polyunsaturated fats such as in fish and flax seed, which both contain important omega-3. Among other benefits, these fats can actually help lower cholesterol levels. The bad fats are saturated and from meat sources and processed foods that are responsible for raising cholesterol levels.

Fat is a slow burning fuel. And healthy fat (those low in hydrogenated oils) helps keep blood sugar levels level. They're fantastic fuel for long-distance efforts (just look at the Chia seeds, made famous by Chris McDougall's *Born to Run* for being the super food of the long-distance Tarahumara). It's no wonder they're filled with quality, slow-burning fat to help keep runners going.

When I was coming back from injury from my broken hip, I was struggling to keep my weight down. I didn't want to get heavy because I wanted to stay light to protect my ailing feet. However, no matter how few calories I ate, and no matter how little fat I ingested, I couldn't get my body fat down. In fact, it went up. Turns out, the less I ate, the more I slowed my metabolism, and the more the body stored energy as fat.

Then I tried what sports nutritionists had recommended for me for years, I increased the fat in my diet, primarily in the form of nuts and oils. Surprisingly, my weight went down, my body fat went down, and my energy levels went up.

As a runner, you may be trying to reduce your weight or maintain. I've never seen as many eating-disordered athletes as in runners, except perhaps among cyclists. Why? Because we all want to keep our weight down to make it easier to move along and go uphill. For us barefoot runners, the less weight we're carrying (at least in body fat not in muscle), the lighter we are on our feet—to a point. Unlike shod runners, we may end up with a little more muscle on our legs—not because we're eating too much, but because we're the support and shock absorbers now, rather than our shoes. But this muscle doesn't slow us down; it makes us lighter on our feet, springier, more resilient, more resistant to injury, and helps us go fast—darn fast! So don't sweat the muscle or the weight. Focus on your health, not on your weight or body fat percentage.

While I don't believe there's an exact ratio that works for everyone, I'd recommend a diet that's higher in protein and fat than we've been told as runners and up to a gram of protein per pound of body weight. I'd say it's more of an Atkins-type diet, except that some people on Atkins go meat or protein crazy, eating meals incredibly high in meat, or stuffing themselves with protein drinks. All this is good for is constipation and killing off your liver—neither of which you want if you're to be healthy for a lifetime.

Fat burns better than any rocket fuel (fancy sports bars and drinks), at least when it comes to long distances. Additionally, it doesn't stimulate your appetite. When you're eating more fat, you only eat when your body's hungry, not when it has an artificially induced sugar craving.

Studies now show fat helps human performance too. We used to think you needed sugar to go fast, but now we're seeing that's only for a pure sprint. Anything below that will still burn a certain amount of fat, and that percentage goes up, the more you train these systems. Unless you're running flat-out, you'll benefit from increasing the fat in your diet—in particular, for long-distance running or training.

Have we had it backwards about fat and carbs all these years?

New studies are now showing what many ultra-endurance athletes have known for years: you can adapt to burning higher quantities of fat, and that it raises VO2, or the amount of oxygen you can consume or burn during high-intensity exercise. In short, fat may improve your performance.

Does this mean go out and load up on Whoppers? No. But it means that eating more healthy fat in your diet will help train your body for distance events and for training, almost no matter what the intensity. Only caveat? You won't be burning fat during your sprints or shortest events, but you can still refuel on a higher fat diet.

Why would you want to do this? Because fat's a more efficient fuel delivery source, it's more natural than stuffing yourself with carbs for hour after hour; it leaves your blood sugar levels closer to normal and, along with protein, acts as more of an appetite suppressant than fast-burning sugary carbs.

Think about this for a mind-bender. You may lose weight (if that's your goal) faster on a higher fat diet than a lower one. Why? Because your body adapts to what it burns. That's why Eskimos can exist and hunt for hours a day (burning as many calories and at as high of an intensity as a warm-weather marathoner) on a nearly pure fat diet. They've trained their bodies to burn fat efficiently for their hunts, even at high intensity levels.

Studies now show that cyclists performed best on time trial tests on a higher fat (70 percent) diet than on a lower fat (30 percent) diet.

So it all comes down to this. If you're doing anything but pure sprints, a higher fat diet may be more healthy for you. And if you're trying to burn fat and get down to whatever you feel is your best weight (I am not an advocate of running around looking like a food-starved anorexic to run at your best), then increase your fat intake. This will help you burn fat more effectively and keep you from craving the sugary carbs.

● °°°₀ FOOT NOTE

- Fat is good for you.

- The higher percentage of fat in your diet, the more you learn to burn fat.

- Burning fat increases endurance, increases VO2 max, and reduces cortisol.

- Eating fat helps you burn fat to lose weight.

- Eating fat helps reduce your appetite.

- Eating fat keeps blood sugar levels steady.

- Eating fat helps you recover more quickly.

Sugar

Years ago coaches used to give their athletes sugar pills before competitions. This was disastrous, as sugar pills would first spike blood sugar levels, then crash them through the floor, leaving athletes listless when they needed energy the most. Today, however, athletes do the same thing, chugging sports-energy drinks before competition loaded with sugars and quick-burning carbs.

When I raced in Europe I learned a trick that's helped me to this day. We learned to race while eating fatty, high-protein foods. We'd eat sandwiches, and rice pudding pies, and all sorts of things you'd never consider "performance" oriented. But in a 3-, 4-, or 5-hour race or longer, these "treats" would save our lives.

The Mind and Diet: Super Foods

When you're running barefoot, you're running more aware—more in touch with your body and the world around you, more tuned in, and less focused on distractions.

To do this, you must keep your mind as properly fueled as your body. If not, you may lose your awareness, and being barefoot, distraction can quickly lead to injury. To keep your mind strong and focused, you must prevent blood sugar crashes (which turn your brains to mush) and keep up the amino acids (fuel for the brain) and essential fatty acids.

This again means more protein and fat. It also means basic brain-food supplements, such as omega-3 fatty acids and fish oils (make sure they're mercury-free).

Additionally, I recommend what I like to call expensive berry juice—or juice from dark-colored berries. The key ingredient is *resveratrol*—a heart-healthy antioxidant found in red wine but also in less-intoxicating juices. Let the food label be your guide. These have been shown to have a positive effect on the brain, as well as being a natural antioxidant (keeping those nasty free radicals at bay), and an anti-inflammatory—perfect for keeping you healthy and aiding with recovery. A few more super foods deserve mention.

Chocolate

To me, chocolate is the greatest super food of the world. Chocolate doesn't just taste great. I first discovered the health benefits of chocolate when working in the ADHD world. Many students and adults were using chocolate to self-medicate or help them calm down and focus. Turns out, the caffeine in chocolate helps those with attention deficit do just that.

Additionally, as a fat from plants, it has amazing antioxidant effects from flavonoids (pigments from plants) that help reduce blood pressure and cholesterol.

Studies show chocolate may have a calming effect and help get your brain in the theta wave pattern, great for brainstorming and idea creation. It also stimulates the release of endorphins, which help you achieve your runner's high and help combat pain and inflammation.

For my morning runs, in particular in the winter, I love having a bit of chocolate (at the same time I'm eating peppers). It helps wake up my mind, allows me to focus, and the slow-burning, healthy fat that's in chocolate helps keep me going.

Spices

Why anti-inflammatory spices? Because they aid in recovery, key to getting you back on the road faster after each workout, and building strong, healthy, happy feet, fast. I'd recommend two natural anti-inflammatory spices (though there are many).

Turmeric, typically used in Indian foods, has a list of positive qualities far too long to list in this book, but as a natural wonder drug, it's a powerful pain killer, anti-inflammatory, anti-cancer, and cleansing food that's safe enough to be taken daily, yet without the harmful effects of anti-inflammatories such as ibuprofen or others.

Cinnamon is another one of those wonder foods. Not only does it have fantastic blood sugar regulatory effects and anti-inflammatory power and apparent amazing benefits in reducing or eliminating pain from arthritis, but is said to warm the feet and increase circulation in people with cold feet.

Hot peppers

To me, this is another natural super food and one of the greatest in the world for barefoot runners. I discovered hot peppers while trying to overcome colds, bronchitis, and my sinus infections. If nothing else, peppers will warm you up and increase your metabolism (and did I mention they are loaded with vitamin C?). For me, if I'm going barefoot on a cold day, then I'm all about eating peppers.

Flax seed oil

Like fish oil, flax seed oil contains healthy omega-3 fatty acids, which are excellent anti-inflammatories, antioxidants, adept at lowering cholesterol, and even shown to be effective at chasing away the blues. Flax seed oil has also been shown to lower triglyceride levels and blood pressure.

Supplements

Although healthy joints and bones are important for all runners, they're particularly important when you can't rely on a shoe.

Runners may want to consider supplements for healthy bones and joints. You might talk with your doctor about a combination of glucosamine, chondroitin, and MSM, which all have many clinical trials showing their benefits for building or rebuilding healthy joints, including aiding cartilage, ligaments, and synovial (joint) fluid.

When selecting supplements (and that includes vitamins), read the list of ingredients on the bottle. You want to see all natural ingredients, a lack of additives, no names you can't read or understand, and no preservatives. Basically, the less "stuff" or additives the better. Also calculate how much of the active ingredient is really in there rather than relying on the misleading front label. For instance, the front label may say 500 IU and 90 pills, so you would assume it's 90 servings of 500 IU. But then if you read the directions it may say, "Take 3 pills per day for 500 IU." Big difference.

Calcium and vitamin D: Even if you think you're getting enough calcium and vitamin D in your diet, you probably are not. Especially in the winter, you can't produce much vitamin D. If you live in Colorado or northern latitudes, the sun's angle is not helpful. That's why most Americans and our children in particular are deficient in vitamin D, which is essential to help our bodies (and bones) absorb calcium.

Vitamin E helps with circulation and anti-arthritic effects, not to mention being kind to the skin. Though its best benefits may be derived topically, vitamin E taken orally is still important for strong healthy, flexible skin (it helps prevent aging of the skin too, and may help prevent skin cancers among other things). It's also said to help with the absorption of vitamin A, which is an important immune system booster.

The B vitamins are the stress busters. If you're under stress, working hard, or running hard, it's important to get your B's. There are many forms of vitamin B, but a complete vitamin B complex may do the job. Vitamin B helps with everything from healthy skin, to good circulation to energy (which is why it's important to take when under stress), sound nervous system function, and much more. While there are many B vitamins, they all work as a team, which is why it's best to take a B-complex vitamin. Additionally, B vitamins are excreted daily in urine, so it's okay to take a relatively high dose (don't be alarmed if it turns your pee bright yellow).

In a perfect world, we would all get the nutrients, including vitamins, we need from food—their natural form—instead of from pills. We just simply don't. You can get as close to the source of natural nutrients by choosing "real foods"—raw, organic, and locally grown.

Better Fuel for Better Running

During the 2009 Leadville 100, I paced Barefoot Ted for 7 hours through the night. Not only did I run alongside him, I carried a heavy 20-pound pack filled with water bottles, food, gels, lights, clothing, and more. My job was to keep him well fueled and hydrated. When running 100 miles, you need proper food and hydration. But what? The delicate balance is different for everyone, but this section gives you a peek into the backpack of the trail runner.

Experts don't agree on the simplicity of this idea, but let me tell you the current thinking.

The faster you run, the more your running is fueled by stored glycogen, and therefore has relatively little to do with what you ate just before a race. The slower you run, the more you tap stored fat for fuel along with carbs and recently eaten foods.

If you're running slower and your objective is to run longer, you might want to consider a mix of faster burning carbs, slower burning carbs, fats and proteins (for example, nut butters and olive oil) to give you a more sustainable energy base for your longer distance runs.

So if you need fuel when you run, what should you do?

Gels, bars, and other munchies

I think people often overeat on runs. Perhaps it's the fear of running out of fuel that gets the better of them. But if you're running less than an hour, it's rare you have to eat. Unless, perhaps, you haven't fed yourself well over the last few days.

But with that said, in long events, or for long training, you may want to eat for a couple of reasons. First of course, to keep yourself well fueled. Second, so that your body is used to eating during runs in case you have a big race coming up or an ultra-event where you'll need to eat on the fly.

Since you never want to test things out in a race, and your body needs time to adapt to anything, it may be best to eat on your training runs. Experiment with these foods and drinks.

Sports drinks tend to be fancy versions of sugar-water with electrolytes. Electrolytes are very important for long or hot-weather runs. They help keep you from hyponatremia, or a lack of salt in your bloodstream, which is far more dangerous than running out of water. It's a common condition too, when runners over-hydrate during events. So these drinks can help. However, they tend to have a very high sugar content.

Look for a sports drink with the slowest burning sugars possible (consult a glycemic index online to help with this) and avoid drinks with any unhealthy corn syrups. Dilute the drink in half. For all my years racing in Europe, I'd fill a tall water bottle with water up to the neck, then fill the rest with Gatorade—or about two-thirds water to one-third sports drink mix. Experiment and see which works best for you, or where you have the most energy without feeling as if you have the "spins" afterward.

Gel packs tend to taste awful, too sweet, and often artificial, yet they can be your lifeline if you're in trouble and facing the dreaded bonks. My advice, test them out before races or long runs and find the ones that fit your palate the best, don't upset your stomach, and keep your blood sugar from being too spiky (I always look for the ones with the lowest glycemic index sugars, such as Cliff Shots, which are made with brown rice syrup).

Many are much too sweet and taste like cake icing—not what you want on a long run. Also realize, once you start taking in sugar (this goes for sports drinks too), you're playing with fire. As long as you keep the carbs coming in, at least every 20 minutes, you'll be fine. But if you have a gel pack and stop, your blood sugar will rise, then fall precipitously, making it worse than if you've had nothing at all. When I'm pacing runners or in a big race, I carry a watch and set an alarm for every 20 minutes after I begin playing with gel packs.

Shot Bloks and other gummy-type food sources are a quick and easy way to get sugars into you and come with a boost of caffeine. For years I've loved Japanese mochi balls for racing. They're like an individually wrapped super-sized gummi bear. Now manufacturers are catching on to the ease of eating gummi's during a long run or race. Since I now rarely use caffeine, even in races, this tends to make me sick. But for most people, caffeine's a good energy boost during a long event, as it helps you burn fat.

Caffeine itself has been shown to help the body burn fat. It has a stimulant effect, particularly if you're not using it all of the time. I used to use caffeine in races before I found I could train my fat systems for greater efficiency. However, while I never take it anymore, it's in many gels, energy-block-type products, and sports bars out there, to help you get the most energy and boost when you need it. I just don't recommend it, because it seems far from natural too me—unless, perhaps, you're getting it directly from a seed, which has fat in it too. Now that's a great one-two punch!

Chia seeds are what the Tarahumara use when they run. Now since I'm known for riding or running with sunflower seeds, nuts, nut butter, or soy products (I've been known to cook and carry zip-locked soy patties, laden with fat and salt for long efforts), Chia seeds sound like an awesome, natural solution to me. They're slow burning, have a good amount of protein, healthy fatty acids, and are supposed to help keep blood sugar levels steady.

Sports bars (and these aren't the places with a bazillion big-screen TVs). I think most sports bars today have gone right off the deep end. They're laden with sugar, either directly to give you energy, or to help hold the things together. This sugar has two problems: First, it can crash your blood sugar. The higher the sugar content and the glycemic index, the more your body throws insulin into the bloodstream to carry the sugar to the muscles, and the lower your blood sugar goes after you eat if you don't keep eating sugar. This can be terrible for training, long-distance events, or for keeping your cool (as it can trigger shakes, anger, or a fight-or-flight response). The second problem with sugar is that sugar begets more sugar. Sugar's that one food that when you eat it, your appetite isn't satiated, but the reverse. The more you eat sweet foods, the hungrier you get.

On a long run, you want to listen to your body as to when to eat. Do not listen to what your food is telling you. Running aware is the secret to barefoot running, and running on sugar eliminates your nutritional awareness.

FOOT NOTE

Always eat before you're hungry and drink before you're thirsty. If you wait until you're hungry or thirsty, you've likely gone too far, and it'll take an extra effort for your body to catch up if you're still out running or doing the work.

What to eat before a race

Since the days of carbo-loading are gone, I recommend you stick with your traditional diet. Feel free to eat more for a day or two before your event, particularly if that helps put your mind at ease, but don't eat to the point of upsetting your stomach. Much better that your body's in its natural, happy, balanced state, rather than out of whack.

Before a long event or training in the heat, however, stay well hydrated, in particular the day and night before. A difference in hydration in the days and day leading up to a challenging run can significantly affect your performance, heat toleration, and ability to handle running at altitude. If you're even thinking of an endurance event at high altitude, such as Leadville, make sure you're extra well hydrated before your event. Just make sure you keep the electrolytes up too.

In the morning of the event, eat a few hours before the race goes off (about 2 and a half hours) to give your body plenty of time to digest before your event. I'd eat whatever you're typically used to in the morning. If it's a short event, you don't have to eat too big if your nerves are getting to you. If it's a longer event, just eat normally. In fact, that's the best rule of all, because whatever's in your stomach isn't likely going to make the difference—that is, as long as you don't upset your stomach or throw things out of whack. I would never recommend gorging before an event, even a marathon or longer.

I never recommend my athletes eat anything within 30 minutes of an event, so they don't spike and crash their blood sugar. If you feel you need something, or if you crave an energy drink such as Red Bull or whatever the latest rocket fuel is, don't drink it until you're on the starting line, less than 5 minutes before an event. This prevents the dreaded sugar crash. Because once you get going, the adrenaline in your veins will settle your blood sugar down. But in general, this last-minute burst isn't necessary.

Fuel your success

If you want to run at your best, then you need to be well fueled. Proper fuel doesn't just give you energy to get going and keep going, but most importantly aids in recovery. For it's recovering from your runs that helps build you stronger and lets you go again.

Nutrition goes beyond getting enough calories into your diet. Good nutrition requires selecting high-quality calories that help the body, rather than hurt it. It's also important to have a well-balanced diet and make sure you're getting enough nutrients and vitamins. How do you know when you've succeeded in a balanced diet? Your body will let you know.

As Deepak Chopra puts it, "The animals in the forest don't have the vaguest notion of what the US Surgeon General said the minimal requirement is for calcium, zinc … Animals don't get nutritional deficiencies or osteoporosis. The only animal, the only species that gets obese is the human species" because we have stopped listening to our bodies.

So, you don't have to go crazy with dozens of supplements. In fact, the all-natural approach is by far the best. Go organic, fresh, local, and stay away from the fishy names, and you'll probably do great. Fuel yourself well and you'll have more fun on your runs!

Nutrition—About My Diet

I used to be a strict vegan. This started before my accident and continued until I met Jessica. Before I became a vegan, I was sick once or twice a year with bronchitis, constantly catching common colds. In the '90s, I was on antibiotics and had two sinus operations to try to kill off chronic sinusitis and the continuous bronchitis infections.

Nothing seemed to work until I changed my diet. Once I became a vegan, all of this went away, and I never got so much as a cold.

Now with Jessica's fantastic cooking, it's been difficult to maintain my vegan ways. However, I still maintain some of the key rules about my former diet, and they're helping me stay healthy and keep the colds at bay.

In this section, I will tell you what I do regarding nutrition and fueling for barefoot running. Again, I caution that I am not a nutritional expert, and I urge you to find the right balance for your lifestyle and barefoot running success.

My diet isn't perfect. Like most other people's it's a work in progress. However, it has improved dramatically over the years, fuels my performance well, and, some say, keeps me young—if only a little.

In general, I eat a higher fat, lower carbohydrate diet, particularly low in simple carbs, sugars, and bleached products. I have no white bread or direct sugar in my diet, and with the exception of fruit, try to eat foods low on the glycemic index.

Years ago I was scared by fat, and worked hard to keep my diet as low fat as possible. However, I think this had a harmful effect, and to this day I'm very sensitive to blood sugar lows.

I do love my greens these days, along with a wide selection of fruits and vegetables, and I live for peppers. I found peppers to be my magic food, along with chocolate—dark chocolate bars and dark chocolate chips for munching (all without dairy). As someone with an ADD-type mind, I found that peppers help calm me and give me great focus (as has been known by Ayurvedic medicine for thousands of years). Hot peppers help raise my metabolism and warm me up before a day's cold run (the fact that peppers are hot literally raises your body temperature).

In the past I took supplements galore. When racing in Europe I would try anything and everything legal to try to improve my performance. Conclusion: none if it worked, but it did create expensive urine.

Now I eat no protein drinks, expensive shakes, gel packs, power bars, or anything of the sort. They're loaded with quick-burning carbs, and I don't want that. Second, I get more than enough protein in a well-balanced daily diet. And unless they're a food source common in nature (did ancient man really run carrying gels), I don't want to put them in my system.

What I do want is more of the good stuff and the natural stuff. This includes omega-3s, some basic vitamins such as B, C, D, and E along with glucosamine, chondroitin with MSM for my joints and calcium because I don't eat dairy.

I eat more omega-3 fatty acids (found in deep sea fish and flax seed oil among others), which have been shown to lower cholesterol and the bad/good ratio, steady blood sugar, and give my brain more power to think.

I stay away from anything corn-syrup based—something I'm convinced ruins your body's ability to regulate blood sugar and may even lead to diabetes. Surprisingly, I don't drink any sports drinks for the very same reason, and if I want fuel on a run, I look to something higher in fat such as nuts or seeds, but not sugary and sweet.

My belief system says that my body (and yours) can manufacture almost anything that it needs. Our brains are the greatest pharmaceutical production facility on the planet. However, it never hurts to make sure you're getting everything you need.

I've been taking B vitamins to fight the "stress" that comes into my life (such as writing this book). I drink berry juice with resveratrol (one favorite drink contains pomegranate juice) to help with inflammation and which has a great calming effect. Turmeric, which I've taken for years and consider one of nature's most amazing wonder drugs, is a natural spice used in Indian food which not only fights inflammation and removes toxins from the body, but helps tremendously with recovery. I've also added ground Saigon cinnamon to my diet—another super food with blood sugar stabilizing effects.

I'm also going back on a "salad in a bottle." For years I took Meta-Greens and loved it. Now I'm trying Juice-Plus, which has the equivalent of 7 pounds of fruits and vegetables in each serving. Study after study suggests this is beneficial for the immune system, recovery, overall health, and perhaps even reducing the effects of aging. All I know is that I crave vegetables and greens, so I might as well include more of them in my diet.

To keep my once-broken joints healthy and strong, I take glucosamine, chondroitin with MSM, which studies show clinically helps build stronger bones, ligaments, and cartilage. I also take calcium since I can't and don't drink dairy products or milk.

My diet's not anything fancy, though surely not the norm. The more natural, raw, and vegan I can go, the better, though I don't claim to be pure vegan (I love my fish and sushi) or anything of the sort. The higher the fat, the better (I love my almond butter), it keeps me light and energized, without my former crashes. And my diet helps me run. I live for running hours on end, dancing in the woods or on the prairie with nature.

Michael's 11 Fuel Rules for Barefoot Running

1. **Go Organic.** I stay organic as much as possible. Even if I'm having meat—and for me this is primarily fish or eggs. By going organic, I stay free of ingesting growth hormones, antibiotics, and pesticides much non-organic foods are laden with these days. I think this tremendously helps in keeping us healthy. I don't know how much we can wash harmful substances off our foods, as they've likely been sprayed since the days they were seeds and pesticides, for example, become a part of our foods.

2. **Free Range Omega-3 Eggs.** When it comes to eggs, I'm opting for those produced by free range hens, because I think the wellness and happiness of the animals is just as essential for the animals' health and for our health as well. I'm also eating eggs high in omega-3, which may be better for the body and mind and helps keep cholesterol levels down.

3. **Wild Caught vs. Farm-Raised Fish.** I'm staying away from farm-raised fish, as they're not a big source of essential fish oils. Furthermore, according to a study published in *Science*, researchers found high levels of PCBs, dioxins, and other contaminants that pose a cancer risk in farm-raised fish as compared to wild caught. I'm also making note of how much fish I eat in general. I don't want to overdo it on the mercury found even in wild caught fish these days (not that any amount of mercury is truly safe).

4. **Microwave Freedom.** I've unplugged from the microwave. Study after study suggests not only that microwave radiation is harmful to our health (just another reason to go out, get grounded, and drain those ions) but chemically alters our food, producing tremendous amounts of free radicals in what we eat.

5. **Just Say No to Fast Food.** I stay away from fast food. In Danny Dreyer's *ChiRunning*, he talks about foods that are low in "Chi" or positive energy. I

have to believe there's very little positive energy in fast foods, no matter how healthy they're touted to be.

6. **No Sports Bars or Sports Drinks.** I stay away from sports bars and sports drinks. To me, the majority of these are too sweet and too synthetic to be any good for me. They're great rocket fuel, but they can make you crash. I hydrate with water.

7. **Corn Syrup Alternatives.** I steer clear of corn syrup. There's no way this can be natural, and in a society that's having diabetes in epic proportions, fructose and the other "oses" can't be good for us. I know after having been off corn syrup, I literally feel sick, weak, and queasy when I eat it. Opt for organic honey, agave (ideal for hypoglycemics or those sensitive to blood sugar lows), or cane juice when possible.

8. **Gluten Free.** I keep the wheat glutens down. There seem to be two foods that make you crave more food when you eat them. First, sugar. Ever notice, the more sugar you eat, the hungrier you get? It's an appetite stimulant, rather than suppressant. Second, glutens. Here too the more baked goods you eat, the more you crave them. Can't eat just one cookie, right? Additionally, many people are either allergic to glutens or find they cause other food allergies to boot. For instance, I've seen people who thought they were allergic to dairy and stopped eating glutens to find they could eat dairy again without difficulty. It's thought that glutens weren't a natural part of our human diet to begin with, and if we didn't evolve to eat it, steer clear.

9. **Colors of the Rainbow.** I'm eating more colors of the rainbow in as many fruits and vegetables as I can, sampling all colors and flavors. By eating all colors and foods that are sweet (rice, cream, and butter, for examples), sour (lemons, yogurt, cheese), astringent (such as beans, lentils, and peas), pungent (horseradish, of course, and peppers and mustard), and bitter (such as green leafy vegetables, spinach, and broccoli), we help assure we're getting a healthy balance of vitamins and nutrients into our diet.

10. **Everything in Moderation.** I shoot for balance. This means trying not to eat too much of any one food. I used to be a creature of habit, eating the same thing in the same amount each day. But that doesn't help me get all the nutrients I need. Instead, if I mix things up, I'm far more likely to get what I need, and naturally.

11. **Eat What You Crave.** Eat what you crave, as long as it's not sugary or full of glutens. Often our cravings, are telling us something. For instance, if you're craving dark leafy greens, then eat them. They're high in calcium and so many other nutrients your body may be craving. When you become more aware,

something that naturally happens as you go barefoot, you find you're more in touch with your body's needs, not just in terms of exercise, but nutrition as well. You may find the more you go barefoot, the less you'll find yourself eating junk.

You don't have to follow all or perhaps any of these rules to stay healthy and happy for barefoot running. But you really are what you eat, so I recommend eating the best, high-quality foods you can. We often take better care of our cars and meet their high octane needs than we do for ourselves. This is a crime. And if we've invested the time and energy into changing our health and our running, then we might as well make the same investment in our fuel choices as well.

You want to be the healthiest you can be, and for a lifetime, right? Then eat right.

⦿°°₀ FOOT NOTE

Because I no longer consume sugar or sugary drinks, sports drinks have not only lost their appeal, but feel bad to me—making me spin and shaky. During a race I may go for a low-glycemic-index gel if I need one, or more likely some Starburst jelly-beans (my favorite if I need sugar on the go), but I tend to stay away from the drinks and instead put water into my system. I might consider the sports jelly-beans, which have electrolytes in them as well. But I want my water to be straight water.

If you want to run at your best, then you need to be well fueled. Proper fuel doesn't just give you energy to get going and keep going, but fuel helps you with the all-important recovery. For it's recovering from your runs that helps build you stronger and lets you go again.

PART III

Dancing with Nature

Climb the mountains and get their good tidings.
Nature's peace will flow into you as sunshine flows into trees.
The winds will blow their own freshness into you ...
while cares will drop off like autumn leaves.

—John Muir

10

Weather or Not, Here I Come

*Sunshine is delicious, rain is refreshing, wind braces us up, snow is exhila-
rating; there is really no such thing as bad weather, only different kinds of
good weather.*

— John Ruskin

Abebe Bikila won the marathon at the 1960 Olympics running barefoot across
pavement and ancient Roman cobblestone roads. He'd trained and conditioned
his feet on jagged dried mud, hot sands, wet mud, and other rugged terrain. And then,
he was ready. With the challenging conditions of the 1960 Olympics, running into
the night on torch-lit roads, I'd say it was because of his bare feet that he won. He'd
been practicing on challenging terrain, and it paid off.

Ancient messengers from Turkey, Tibet, Peru, and all through North America ran
hundreds of miles at a time nonstop. Sherpas climb the high Himalayas in nothing
but a pair of sandals. To this day, Aborigines run barefoot through hot desert sands.
And island children run on razor-sharp coral reefs without a single scratch.

I'm known for wearing a full track running suit at 90 degrees to adapt to the heat,
and shorts below freezing to adapt to the cold. I'll run on gravel roads to strengthen
my feet, and on loose mountain trails to help improve my balance. All of these un-
conventional training methods help and have allowed me to do some fun stuff, but
these physical adaptations are nothing compared to what we can do with our minds.

It helps to know the best ways to get into the fun stuff. And by fun, I mean the
most challenging surfaces, temperatures, and conditions you can think of. Although

I don't see barefoot running as an extreme sport, our ancestors did it just for basic survival.

Let's look at the major challenging conditions out there, from heat to cold and rain to snow; from different road conditions, trail conditions, and other hazards to watch out for—and the gear to best prepare you for a rocky road ahead.

Like it or not, the roads aren't always smooth, the trails aren't always soft, and it's not always spring. But you can prepare for the best and the worst and be the strongest, most well-balanced runner, capable of handling all that comes your way.

How Cold or Hot Is It?

Air temperatures can be quite deceiving. Even though it may be a pleasant, sunny 60-degree day, that doesn't guarantee your running surfaces (manmade or natural) are going to be just as warm and pleasant. (All temperatures here are expressed in Fahrenheit.) If the 60-degree day is a "fluke" in the dead of winter, chances are likely the ground is still holding onto a freezing temperature.

Not all surfaces are created equal, denser/harder surfaces are slower to cool and slower to heat. So there's quite a number of factors to consider when you're gauging ground temperature, such as the temperature of previous days, humidity levels, and surface material.

All temperatures are not equal. Running at 32 degrees with humidity—which leads to things freezing—makes the ground substantially colder than without humidity. And the ground is a lot colder after 5 days of 32-degree temps than on the first near-freezing day.

Ground temperature has a much bigger impact on your feet than air temperature, so forget about weather reports and pay the most attention to how your feet feel. Different surfaces (ice, snow, cement, asphalt, mud, brush) drain away more heat from your feet. For instance, wet snow takes away more heat than dry snow, and wet mud sucks away heat even faster than moist snow. Wet pavement (such as asphalt, which some people think of as blacktop) also takes away more heat than dry pavement.

Pavement and cement are slow to cool off (cement seems to hold its temperature better, but once it's cold, due to both color and density it's far colder than the blacktop), but if you've had a good cold spell, or the cold's set in for the season, then even on a warmer winter's day, the ground temperature may be far colder than the air.

Different surfaces also hold different amounts of heat. For example, pavement, ice, and wet conditions can be deceiving, particularly depending on recent sunlight. Sometimes the ice next to the bright-colored sidewalk is warmer than the sidewalk itself. Blacktop, even if wet, may be warmer than a lighter colored surface. And if there's snow melt in your path, the wet surface may be warmer than the dry one you're trodding on. Final point, sometimes the ice you're trying to avoid may be much warmer than the cold cement you're jogging on. There's an art to determining which surfaces let your feet stay the warmest. Try the different surfaces and different conditions and see what works best.

Hot surfaces can be tricky as well. On any given day, pavement and cement are likely two very different temperatures, and trails far different than both. Cement heats up gradually over time, then cools off gradually as well, while pavement heats up fast, then quickly sheds its heat. Trails are another story entirely, depending on the dirt, dryness, and rock beneath. Make note of this, and run head's up so you don't get burned. Extreme conditions are never to be taken casually.

Running in Heat: Concrete Advice

Since you can't always choose where or when to run, it's best to prepare for as many conditions as possible. If you're running in the summertime, unless you do it pre-dawn, chances are you'll have some baking-hot-asphalt days. But not to worry, a hot tarmac can actually be a good thing. No other condition helps temper and strengthen your feet like hot stone.

Humans may have adapted naturally for this in the past. According to evolutionary biologists, we first became erect and began running in the hot African savannah. This may explain why our feet adapted so well to the heat. It strengthens our skin and increases padding, increases circulation, aids foot strength, and more.

Adapting to running in the heat

Heat helps in many ways. First and foremost, it stimulates pad growth more than anything else. This additional padding helps you handle the heat and rough surfaces. In essence, you're growing stronger "shoes" in the summertime. This will benefit you in all conditions year round.

You're increasing circulation to your feet. Your body adapts and increases capillaries and blood flow to your feet to help keep your feet cool and strong, and for recovery. After a great run in the heat, or even in the cold, your feet will remain hot at night. This isn't because they're burning, but because of the extra blood your body's pumping to your feet to rebuild and grow your padding stronger. This increased blood flow will help your feet and your padding in the summer, and help keep your feet warmer in the winter too. And there's another tremendous benefit. Increased blood flow means

◉°°°₀ FOOT NOTE

Always bring your shoes with you. When your feet feel too hot, don't think twice, put them on. I like to say put your shoes on before your feet feel too hot, and before they feel too cold, because by the time they feel too hot or too cold, you've likely gone too far or done too much.

shorter recovery times, both for normal recovery from a hard workout—and in case you overdo it. Increased blood flow helps ligaments, tendons, and even bones recover faster.

Although hot conditions are ideal for pad development, they can be quite dangerous too. Heading out in the heat before you're ready could leave you badly burned, or with blistered feet that look like pepperoni pizza.

Whether you're a beginner or expert, once spring rolls around, you want to baby your feet into the heat. While heat may stimulate growth and improve circulation, it requires significant time for feet to recover.

Transitioning into hot weather

Once the heat hits, follow these weekly steps to keep from cooking your feet and helping them learn to sizzle:

- Week 1: When it gets hot, skip the midday runs for a week or so, and instead go out for short walks. This helps temper your feet and keeps you close to home. Always walk with hand weights (shoes) and never think twice about putting them back on.

- Week 2: Venture out jogging for short distances, perhaps a half mile to a mile at most.

- Week 3 and after: Go longer in the heat and add one long run a week for the first month or two.

The worst thing you can do is go out in the heat two days in a row (or in the winter, out in the cold two days in a row). While your feet are growing back stronger, the day after a hot run your feet have temporarily lost their resistance to the heat. Your skin's now soft, your padding mush, and you'll burn yourself extraordinarily fast. This is also why I recommend only one extra-long run in the heat a week for the first month or two. The additional distance requires additional time to recover. After a long Saturday run in the heat, I won't touch the stuff for several days, and then do short hot runs until the weekend again.

One of the best ways to transition to the heat is to alternate between hot and cool surfaces on your run, such as hopping between a blacktop road and a sidewalk. You can do this for 100 yards at a time, or however long your feet can handle letting the heat be your guide. Never push too much or too far. If your feet start cooking, head back onto the cool stuff. By alternating, you let your feet cool down between efforts. It's the long steady heat that'll cook them.

Warning signs

During my first time transitioning to heat, I didn't heed the warning signs. I knew when it was time to come home, my feet were getting soft and tender. But I thought to myself, *I'll just do one more mile, then head for home.* Well, that mile was the killer, a slightly abrasive blacktop surface that finished off my pads and developed two heat blisters. The good news is, the pads grew back stronger than ever in those areas. The bad news: there was no reason to abuse my feet in that way. When your pads feel soft, start to get too hot, or just don't feel right, slip on those shoes and head for home.

I also recommend heading out on hot rocky or sandy trails in the heat if you can get your feet on them. Here in Boulder, we have a very steep, rocky trail with smooth large granite stones for clambering. It really heats up in the summer, but the three-dimensional texture of the stones helps build strong pads. I've also heard the sand dunes in southern Colorado are great for tempering feet. There's likely some similar conditions near you too.

When I head out in the heat, even after I've transitioned, I'm always looking for routes where I can find shade if necessary. Road temperatures can easily be 10 to 20 degrees cooler or more in the shade. Not to mention the air being cooler as well when out of the sun. Look for routes that offer protection if you need it. You might spot trees along the side of the road, a way back through the trees on a trail, or even in the shade of nearby buildings. Shade's another way to extend your run and keep you safe.

There's an amazing race in California called the Badwater Ultra-marathon. It runs 135 miles nonstop from Death Valley to Mount Whitney where temperatures can approach 130 degrees (55 degrees Celsius). There are other races around the world across the Sahara and other flaming hot deserts. Athletes must be prepared for the most extreme conditions. Tempering your feet for the heat can help.

Water, water, too much water

When it comes to hydration, think safety first. What I'll say next should be done with extreme caution.

When running in the heat, if you're well prehydrated you may not need as much water, or water as often as you think. I see so many runners out there with a water bottle in hand, chugging it down every 5 minutes or so right from the start. First, if you're running with only one bottle, there's no way to stay balanced, and that's a problem. Second, you likely don't need as much water as you think, at least in the short run, according to Timothy Noakes, a South African physician who wrote a definitive guide on technical running, called *The Lore of Running*.

According to many recent studies, the bigger danger when running in the heat may be drinking too much, rather than not drinking enough. It's hypothesized that we did long hunts in the hot savannah heat without any water and that our bodies adapted to handle this stress.

Overwatering, or a term called *hyponatremia*, is quite common in endurance events.

A study at the 2002 Boston Marathon found 13 percent of the 488 participants to be hyponatremic, and 2 of those dangerously so. In a three-year study of the Houston Marathon, a staggering 28 percent of participants were found to be hyponatremic after finishing.

Too much water is a real danger, and a tricky one. I helped pace Barefoot Ted for the last 26 miles of the Leadville 100 in the summer of 2009. When he came to me, his pace was slowing and he seemed a bit weak. It'd been an incredibly hot day for the race, and many participants were dehydrated or overheating. I didn't know how much water he'd drank, nor how many salt tablets he'd swallowed, nor even how much food he'd eaten in the previous 74 miles.

I helped Barefoot Ted rehydrate, but without knowing how much he'd been drinking, nor how much salt, or food, was in his system, I didn't have the information I needed to prevent over-watering. At the end he finished strongly, but was borderline hyponatremic. It just goes to show, even the best of us can be tricked, and you must learn your body well.

In addition to the danger of over-watering, carrying water might mess up your stride. If you don't need the water, but it's only a mental thing, consider cutting back on the water, or holding off for a bit. Yes, there's a big concern with dehydration and the heat, but it's very unlikely that'll happen in a 20- or 30-minute run.

If this is something you'd like to explore, I recommend starting out on hot days with short runs (10 to 20 minutes) without water and building up from there. Your body can likely handle several hours in the heat without water, if you build in slowly and teach your body to adapt.

Prehydrate

To begin to train yourself and understand how your body reacts with proper prehydration, drink lots of extra fluids the night before a hot run and just prior to the hot run. How much? Drink as much as you can to where you won't be stopping every 5 minutes off the side of the road to pee. Additionally, don't drink so much you can't run because water's sloshing around in your belly. You'll have to find the exact amount that works for you through trial and error or feel.

Then start out with 20 or 30 minutes in the heat without water. Recover a few days before attempting it again. Then go for just 5 or 10 minutes more. Build up from here gradually, but always play it safe. No matter what, bring some water in a hydration pack (not in a water bottle held in one hand) when you're just starting out and getting to know your body in the heat. If you start to wonder if you made a smart decision, get yourself home, to the shade, or your car fast.

The body's amazing at adapting, but this is one area where you want to be exceptionally careful. Native Americans and other persistence hunters around the world have trained their bodies to go hour after hour in the hot desert heat without water and seemingly without sweating. But they started slowly; if not, they wouldn't be around to tell the tale.

Less bounce to the ounce

When the going gets hot, and you need water along, look for a hydration pack that doesn't affect your stride. Basic hydration packs often bounce on your back. This bouncing affects everything about your rhythm and stride. Look for a pack that keeps the water low on your belt (Inov-8 has a new series that keeps the water down by your waist such as the Inov-8 Race Pro series).

The lower your center of mass, the better it is for your stride. A hydration belt may work well too, but just make sure it doesn't affect your stride, arm movement, or your shoulders or back. In short, make sure it doesn't affect your center of gravity or alignment.

As with any new change in gear (even with socks) build up your new time with your gear slowly and tinker to find just the right position. Often a change of one inch in height up or down of your pack can be the difference between staying healthy on your toes and coming down midfoot and crushing your foot over time. Work to find the sweet spot and make sure, no matter what pack you get, it has a waist strap to keep it from bouncing.

Running in Cold:
Enough to Freeze Your Tootsies Off

Now that your feet are hot and sweaty, let's take a look at the other side of the coin. Your body not only adapts to heat amazingly well, but to extreme cold too. Again, you have to start slow, more slowly than you ever imagined. But if you do, then you too may be the next Ice Man, running snow and ice with ease, amazing yourself even more than your friends.

It turns out, wearing an over-supportive shoe or boot shunts blood flow away from your feet. When your shoe does the work for your foot, your foot muscles relax, and blood flow is diverted to other muscles in your body performing more work. It's the lack of blood flow to the feet that causes them to cool. When you're going barefoot, the muscles in your feet are forced to work hard to support you and keep you going. So instead of blood flow shunted away from your feet and to other parts of the body, your body starts delivering more blood to your feet.

When you run barefoot in the cold, you'll see your feet start to turn beet-red from increased blood flow. In fact, my feet tend to be hot and sweaty for hours after a cold winter's barefoot run.

For myself, the first few weeks in the cold are the most difficult, and then I'm far more comfortable. However, I'm still careful in mid-winter snows because the ground is far colder than in the fall or the spring.

Adapting to cold-weather running

As with other aspects of running bare, you should build up your foot tolerance to cold very gradually. A good approach is to run on a path close to your home or gym, so when you feel your feet getting cold despite the blood your body is pumping to them, you can hurry inside and warm them up ASAP.

With late autumn come the season's first few frosts. Warm up your feet well, either by starting in shoes, a few minutes running stairs, or walking on a treadmill, then head on out. Run where it's dry and keep this first run short and close to home. The minute your feet start getting cold, don't think twice, put on your shoes and get home fast. Just like the heat, it's important to cool off before your feet feel too hot, and warm them up before they ever feel too cold.

Just as with the heat, never go two days in a row, but measure your progress. If, on your last run, your feet made it 10 minutes before getting cold, consider an extra minute your next day out. Running every other day, or even every third day, will build your feet up much faster than daily runs. Also note the temperature. If it's 30 degrees one day and you go for 20 minutes, and the next time it's 20 degrees, don't expect to go as far. In fact, perhaps only 5 minutes the next time is all that's safe.

As you continue doing this week after week, you'll find that it's taking longer and longer before your feet grow cold. That's because your pads adapt and your body is learning to pump increasingly more blood to them. For example, I can run bare on snow for hours, but it took years of training for my body to reach this point.

Oddly, ice can be warm, at least relative to the air temperature. Get good at cold weather runs and you'll see what I mean. If ice on your path is near 32 degrees and a hard frost has the ground at 10 degrees, it may be warmer running ON the ice. Or ice on frozen blacktop may be warmer than the white cement bike path it parallels. These are just a few of the mind-benders you'll find when exploring winter terrains.

You may also notice that snow melt is the warmest place to run. This is another mind-bender, but be careful with this one. We're not too worried about wearing the pads, they get harder in the cold, but if there's any rock salt in that snow melt, then lookout—your pads could be gone in a minute. Rock salt acts like a meat tenderizer, and you're the roast.

⦿°°₀ FOOT NOTE

Strange as it seems, you may have more traction with your bare feet on ice than with your shoes. It depends on the heat and humidity, and how much sweat the glands on your feet produce. But often our feet become like Spiderman's—grippy little suction cups hold the ice when we run. Just make sure you stay on your toes. The more pounds per square inch you put down, and the more you put your weight forward, the less likely you are to slide.

Dirt trails in the winter pose a unique challenge. With different shade, surfaces, and rocks, they're often incredibly unpredictable. I'd start on the manmade surfaces long before you head for the trails, and when you do, bring some exceptionally warm footwear with you. Personally, I carry my neoprene moccasins as well as hand-warmer packs (iron-filled packs that oxidize and heat up when exposed to the air). An eco-friendly option are Wonder Warmers, heat packs that recharge when you boil them.

When you're on the paths and roads, you know what's coming and can get home fast, but out on the trails, you're in a different world, an unpredictable one, filled with more great challenges, requiring exceptional caution.

Even though your skin may be strong in the cold, your muscles, tendons, and ligaments won't be as supple. Warm your feet up well and then ease into uneven terrain with extreme caution. Your feet lose their flexibility in the cold unless they're incredibly warmed up and you keep your speed up. This means you're more susceptible to overuse injuries, tripping, or even rolling an ankle. Just another reason to keep to the flat stuff or exceptionally mild terrain until you know your body well and become an experienced winter-weather barefoot runner.

The skin of your feet is less pliable and therefore often feels stronger in the cold. This makes them better suited for many conditions, but more sensitive to the little things. Since the skin is less flexible in the cold, you may find yourself more sensitive to little pebbles and other small obstructions. Be on the lookout.

Snowtocol—Protocol for Running in the Snow

Interested in trying out the fluffy stuff for yourself? Here's a checklist to get into the snow without getting burned.

- **Warm-up First.** Consider running stairs, a treadmill, or starting out with your shoes on. Warming up not only keeps your body warm, but keeps your feet warmer and more limber in the snow. Cold, stiff feet on snow get injured when you try to flex them. You need warm, flexible, relaxed feet, before you hit the fluffy stuff. If you make sure you're just about breaking a sweat before you head out, then you know your body's ready.

- **Run from Your Home or the Gym.** Don't start your run from your car. Instead, begin from somewhere where you can warm up fast, such as your home or a fitness center with a treadmill.

- **Begin with a Few Minutes at Most.** Warm up, then do 3 to 5 minutes outside, then 3 to 5 minutes back indoors again, such as on a treadmill or running up and down your stairs. If you feel good, head back out and repeat. You can do this until your feet stay too cold when you get back indoors; when that's the case, you're done. This approach lets you test your feet and the limits, without going into the danger zone.

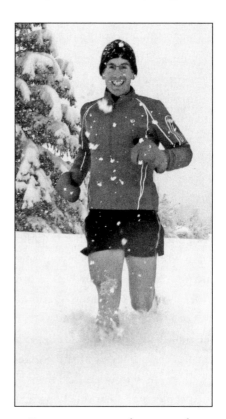

- **Stay on Your Toes.** There are 3 reasons why staying on your toes keeps your feet warm: (1) Works your foot more, therefore the body must deliver more warm blood to the foot. (2) Leaves less contact area with the cold ground. (3) Focuses more weight on a smaller area of your foot, giving you greater traction and allowing you to grip with your toes. Never run flat-footed or on your heels even in soft snow, or you will slip, slide, and fall.

- **If You Feel the Heat—Head for Home.** If your feet start to burn or get numb, head for home. If they're fully numb, this does NOT mean they're doing well, it mean's they're cooked, get inside, NOW.

Running even in deep snow becomes possible, if not fun, after you've trained your body for the cold. Michael runs through 18–20 inches of powder during an early Colorado snowstorm.

- **Layer-up Your Upper Body.** Don't dress like the Michelin Man, but plan on at least an extra layer or two over what you'd wear in dry conditions in the cold. The warmer your upper body, the less your feet will have to work to keep warm.

- **Wear Unrestrictive Clothing.** Restrictive clothing reduces circulation and quickly cools you off fast. It can also affect your stride, making you slow, cumbersome, and prone to injury. The more you move freely, the faster, happier, and warmer you'll be.

- **Wear a Hat—or Two.** Up to 80 percent of all body heat is lost through your head, so cover it up. I have made the mistake of heading out without a hat in the snow before. Though I'd done the distance and the snow many times, I was foolish to go out without a hat. I almost got in severe danger before finding a way to stay warm. Always wear a hat or even two when running in the cold, let alone in the snow.

- **Always Wear Gloves and Consider Hand-warmers Too.** Unlike your feet, which will be doing a lot of work, your hands get precious little warm blood flow. Wear warm gloves, and consider hand-warmers. The warmer your hands, the warmer your feet. If you freeze your hands, your toes will soon follow.

- **Watch for Rock Salt.** Salt is also used to tenderize meat—and unfortunately it has the same effect on your feet by rapidly softening the pads you've worked so hard to build up. I've only been cut by glass once—on a salty sidewalk during a snowstorm. The sharp rock salt tenderized my feet, and then I ran over something I assumed was just salt.

The power of meditation

Last spring, we went out on a hike to take photos in the mountains around 10,000 feet. We stopped by a lake filled with fresh snow runoff and surrounded by snow. There, in the 32-degree water, I waded out to shoot photographs of surrounding 14,000-foot peaks for 40 minutes. Oddly enough, although I should have been hypothermic or dead, I never got cold.

I attribute this to the power of meditation.

The Lung-Gom-Pa, the mystical group of Tibetan running monks, were capable of going into freezing lakes in the winter and generating enough heat through their meditation that steam would soon rise from their bodies.

Meditation is a way to heat up your body on even the coldest of runs. This can be done while running, or in a quiet setting for practice.

> ### *Exercise:* Meditation
>
> **Try this:** Start by quieting your mind and letting your thoughts drop away. Focus on your breath, taking deep diaphragmatic inhalations and exhalations. With each exhalation, let more of your thoughts fall away.

Once your mind is quiet, visualize the flame of a hot-air balloon burning in the center of your body. Picture your body as a balloon and begin to turn up the burner. With each exhalation, turn up the flame and see your body begin to glow red. As the flame grows, picture the flame generating incredible heat throughout your entire body.

Block out all thought and focus simply on your breath and the flame. Inhale, envisioning your body warming. Then exhale, watching the flame grow bigger. As you do this, you may witness your skin getting redder as your body begins to rise in temperature.

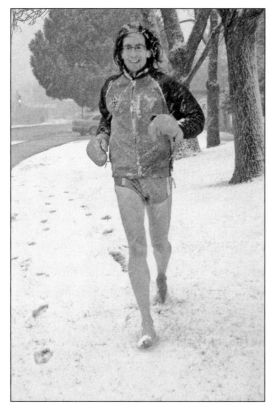

Michael uses the Lung-Gom-Pa meditation technique to keep his feet and legs beet red and hot despite 5K running in a snowstorm.

Don't get bitten: Signs of frostbite

- Gradual numbness and loss of touch

- Tingling or burning sensation

- A feeling as if your hands or feet are wood

- Associated pain that then goes away (as the frostbite progresses)

- Change in the color of your hands or feet from pinkish-red to blanched, white, or white-purple (or far worse, black)

If you think you have frostbite, get inside quickly. Warm things up fast. I recommend warming up your feet fast under 104- to 105-degree water if you got cold fast. Don't go too hot, because you won't be able to tell what's scalding and what's not. But ignore the old wives' tale that you need to warm things up slowly. The general rule among winter emergency specialists is this: freeze fast, thaw fast and freeze slow, thaw slow (an example of slow freezing would be on an Everest expedition).

If there are signs of discoloration after fingers and toes, ears and other parts have been heated up, you should see a doctor. Wrap the affected area in loose bandages (warning: tight bandages might tear off and injure tissue when removed) and soft clothing to keep it warm and protected, then get to your ER.

If you're stuck out in the cold, the worst thing you can do is warm things up if there's a chance of getting frostbite again. Instead drag yourself to a place where you can get warm and stay warm. Refreezing injured feet always results in far more severe damage. (This is one of the biggest no-no's in survival books out there. Never let things refreeze.)

Do not rub your hands or feet to warm them up *after* they've been frostbitten. This can damage your skin and frozen tissue underneath.

> *I frequently tramped 8 or 10 miles through the deepest snow to keep an appointment with a beech-tree, or a yellow birch, or an old acquaintance among the pines.*
>
> —Henry David Thoreau

People say once you've been frostbitten your hands or feet will always be cold. This is incorrect. Running barefoot not only brings more blood flow to your feet when running in the cold, but over time increases vasculature and perfusion of the entire foot. Your feet become better nourished, have greater warm blood pumping through them, and develop greater insulation in the form of fat and muscle to handle the cold.

No matter how much you adapt your feet to the conditions, there may still be times you need to wear footwear, particularly if you're in a snowy climate. A barefoot running approach to this is simple: look for footwear that offers minimal (or no) support with maximum flexibility.

Cold-weather gear

I've been experimenting with many types of products and there are many more to go. So far, my favorite is to wear a cycling bootie with an insulated Toasty Feet insole beneath. It's the shape and flexibility of a moccasin, which lets your feet move freely and do the work, and the neoprene and insole keep your foot well insulated. If you go the bootie route, make sure they're lightweight, and you start into them slowly (in case it changes your stride). Avoid scuba-diving booties and other similar wet-weather or water gear, as they tend to be tight and form-fitting, which not only leaves your toes unable to move, but reduces circulation.

My neoprene solution seems to be a great way to go in the snow, a bit less so on the dry stuff (particularly when going fast) and not so great on smooth, slick ice. If the terrain is pure ice, consider other footwear with a strap-on traction device (I prefer those with magnesium spikes rather than cables or chains) or wear track spikes inside your booties with cut-outs for the spikes. (I like my Asics Dirt Dogs, but recommend getting extra-long screw-in spikes.)

For either of these options, make sure your circulation is not restricted, and try things out slowly. It's all too common for new runners to have so much fun in the fluffy stuff or ice the first day (without being used to the gear or change in stride and force), they're out of the game for weeks. Realize it inherently changes your stride and feel for the ground (in other words, how hard you strike), so keep the reins tight and start slow.

For extra cold days, I'll always have a couple of what I call tea bags or hand-warmers with me. These are $1 or $2 packets you can pick up at your favorite sports store or grocery (or find eco-friendly, reusable packs called Wonder Warmers). They're handy for emergencies or if you have a hunch things might get cold. Open the packages before they are needed as they take up to 20 minutes to warm up. Once the warmers are exposed to oxygen, they begin to heat up. Hand-warmers can be life-savers when out in the cold or out on the trail. They are often rated to last for 7 to 14 hours. You can reuse them repeatedly up to their rated time if you place them in air-free zipper bags and keep them in your freezer.

⦿°°° FOOT NOTE

Magic Fuel for Keeping Warm

If you want the ancient secret to staying warm in the cold, this is it. According to Ayurvedic medicine, Native American medicine, and other traditions around the world, it's peppers. Any food that makes you sweat not only tastes hot, but literally raises your body temperature and helps keep your feet warm. Peppers also have the added benefit of raising your metabolism by up to 15 percent (not that you need to burn any more calories, but if you do, it may be a worthy idea). The more calories your body burns, the more heat it produces too. So whether you're trying to get in shape or stay in shape, peppers can be a magic fuel. Peppers also pack more vitamin C antioxidants than oranges.

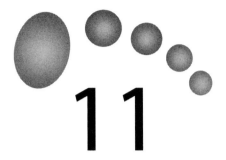

11

Exploring Terrain

And the end of all our exploring
Will be to arrive where we started
And know the place for the first time.

—T.S. Eliot

I f the world were flat, fully paved, and always 70 degrees, it'd truly be a dull place indeed—and a poor place for a foot that thrives on challenge and change. Fortunately, different conditions, temperatures, and surfaces abound. As barefoot runners, we're truly three-dimensional, since we can feel far more than in shoes. This makes varying conditions much more interesting—and challenging.

We're hard-wired for adventure; specifically, for running trails at full speed while hopping from rock to rock. Our ancestors ran for the hunt and for pure joy. When you're running in shoes, every surface seems similar, but there are many different types of surfaces, each with its own unique challenges, characteristics, and requirements. There's almost an unlimited variety of paved surfaces and trails from smooth to rocky and steep to flat. When you're in a shoe, your normal runs may seem dull; but take yourself out of a shoe, and it's a whole new world.

Once you get into challenging terrain, you'll learn something fascinating about yourself. Our minds are capable of looking ahead, looking beneath us, helping us choose a path, and dancing over roots, under branches, and just about anywhere we want—completely connected to the trail and world around us, and yet with a silent mind. There's something incredibly natural, stimulating, and soothing about dancing through the woods, and over many other types of terrain.

In this section we'll examine different surfaces, what to avoid and what to seek out. We'll also look at the ups and downs of uphills, downhills, and mountain running.

The Benefits of Exploring Terrain

It is a rough road that leads to the heights of greatness.

—Seneca

When you feel the ground, you're truly all-terrain (you become your own ATB All-Terrain-Barefoot vehicle). You sense and adjust to conditions instantly. Landing on the ball of your foot allows you to skip a step or lift back up if you need to, in order to avoid rocks, glass, or other obstacles. You could never do that in a shoe, and when you're tired in a shoe, you're likely to trip and stumble over the humblest of obstacles.

With as many nerve endings in your feet as you have in your hands and genitals, your feet feel *everything* on the ground. In the beginning you may think you don't want to feel things, because that tiny little pebble hurts. But over time the pain dissipates. You never want to stop feeling things, because it's the secret to your success. Over time you learn to feel the pebble and make minute adjustments that save you from discomfort. Your feet also learn to relax over the pebble, which spreads out the force too, which greatly reduces discomfort. Your feet learn to react to the ground and any challenges automatically. You'll notice your foot rolled a little to accommodate one rock, landed light to handle another, or even jumped to the side a hair to prevent the ankle twisting that inevitably would have occurred in shoes.

Like a rabbit on crack, you become light, agile, and super-nimble too. You can also adjust your stride length for maximum efficiency. You're not locked into a groove, swinging a heavy boot around. In a shoe you could never jump to the side, midstride. I consider bare feet the most technologically advanced guidance system in the world.

Exercises

The Monkey Jog

What do you do when you hit a surface your pads, feet, and technique aren't ready for? It's simple, drop your landing gear. When it comes to rough terrain and surprises, nothing beats what I call "doing the Monkey Jog." When you begin trails or rough surfaces, you may find some surfaces particularly challenging. This could be your first trail, or first rocky one, a metal grated bridge, a chip and seal stretch of road, or the rockiest downhill of your life.

Try this: To drop your landing gear, you'll simply lower your feet to where your heels are just above the ground. You'll still land on your forefoot, albeit just barely, and instead of rebounding ahead, you'll use your hamstring for propulsion as you push off behind you. You'll drop your arms too, keeping them loose, but bringing them straight down by your sides.

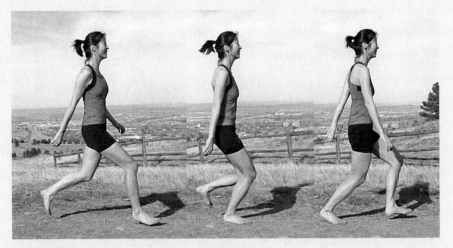

Monkey Jog: Jessica lowers her center of gravity and gets low to handle running on challenging terrain. This reduces bounce and impact and dissipates the force of any sharp, unyielding objects or surfaces.

What you're doing by lowering your feet and landing gear is threefold. First, you're lowering your center of gravity to give yourself more balance. Second, you're putting down more of the foot to give yourself more surface area to spread out the force of the sharp or difficult objects. And third, by lowering yourself, keeping your arms down, and pushing off behind you, you're staying closer to the ground, reducing impact on sharp objects while greatly aiding in stability.

In essence, rocks don't feel as hard or as sharp if you're not bouncing up and down on top of them, but instead almost shuffling along. This lets you keep up the pace (an especially good technique for long runs or ultra-endurance events), while getting you off the rough stuff. It's also a way to rest your quads and calves if you need to.

The Ape Walk

Barefoot Ted's an amazing guy. If you ever get a chance to meet him or attend a clinic of his, I'd highly recommend it. He's very inspirational and I had the honor of pacing him during the last 26 miles of the 2009 Leadville 100.

One thing I noticed while pacing Ted is his amazing ability to walk fast.

Maybe that's an understatement, but while he's walking, he's passing runners around him. When the going got tough and Barefoot Ted needed to walk, he barely slowed down, walking at a pace most jogged, if not ran. By keeping his center of gravity low and pushing off behind him, he was more efficient and passing runners even on the toughest of terrain wearing Vibram FiveFingers footwear.

Getting low helps you get over things easier, gives you better balance, and allows you to use more surface area to handle jagged rocks without pain. It also produces an amazing stride length, which is why Barefoot Ted's walking pace is as fast as many people's jog.

Ape Walking and the Monkey Jog let you get into rougher terrain, which stimulates pad growth and development.

Try this: This technique not only allows you to traverse the most challenging of surfaces, but by helping you do the tough stuff, helps build stronger feet and padding in the process. The next time you're on gravel or something particularly challenging, rather than put on the shoes, use it as a chance to experiment and build your strongest pads ever. Tighten that core, snap your belly button to the back, have that string pull you toward the heavens, squat down low, relax the feet, and be the best monkey you can.

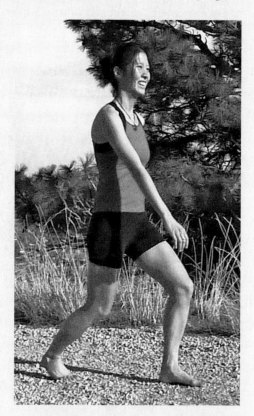

Ape Walk: Similar to the Monkey Jog yet at a walking pace, staying low helps you traverse the most challenging of terrain.

Ski-Walking

Want a new barefoot workout as you're easing into things? Try walking as if you're cross-country skiing. This is best accomplished on a good uphill grade, though it can be done on level ground as well.

> **Try this:** Walk, preferably uphill, imagining your feet are attached to skis. After you grab with your toes with each step, push your skis off behind you to propel yourself forward. Make sure you keep your core tight and upper body steady, without leaning forward or twisting to either side. Your arms can be down by your side, swinging with each stride (like you're doing when Monkey Jogging). But don't concentrate on the arms, let your hand weights do the work (remember those shoes you're carrying with you?) and instead, focus on minimal excess movement.
>
> The goal of this exercise is to push with the legs behind you. It builds hamstring strength while working your core muscles, arches, and every muscle of your feet.

Navigate the Roads Less Traveled

Not all roads are created equal. A shod runner's assessment of a road condition is likely vastly different from a barefoot runner's take. Both Jessica and I noted the difference in perspective in two races we ran. In the first, the course was noted to be easy and soft. That sounded great for us. Turns out, it began on loose gravel (with plenty of cactus on the sides ... ouch) before proceeding to torn-up old pavement on a bike path, and then finishing on chip and seal roads. While shod runners didn't notice the chewed up course, we were deeply humbled.

Then during a local Turkey Trot 5K, we had a similar experience: a smoother chip and seal road that made it difficult to keep up with the group. Personally, I sprang past my fellow runners each time there was a smooth patch, or a cement gutter to run in, but each time I was stuck on the chip and seal, I had to lower the landing gear.

When you're in shoes, it's rare you understand or pay attention to the surfaces beneath you. Sure, if you're doing the miles, you're probably trying to stay off cement as much as possible, and you're probably trying to hit patches of dirt next to cement to keep it soft as well. But you're probably not looking at the ground that closely.

Yet when you go barefoot, you become a student of your terrain. When you're barefoot, you'll find which roads are smooth, which are rough, which have sharp jagged edges, and which are slick. You'll understand the cushion beneath each surface, come up with favorites, and find those best left alone.

Let's explore some of the roads less traveled and discuss how to run them.

Smooth cement bike paths

This is the easiest surface for beginners, but not a favorite over the long haul. The smoothness makes them easy, and the surface gives tremendous feedback. It helps you feel the ground, learn to stride light, and work on your form. However, cement paths have several major challenges.

First, they're likely the hardest surface you'll ever run on—and completely unforgiving. Second, they're flat, perfectly flat. That means there are no undulations, imperfections, or changes on the surface that give your feet a chance to rest and recover, flex, and get proper blood flow. Think of it this way: In nature, we never ran on perfectly flat surfaces. Surfaces changed, sloping one way, then another, getting rough, getting smooth, getting soft, then hard again. These constant changes allowed our feet to recover.

On the trails, if you overwork muscles on the smooth stuff, don't worry, you'll work different muscles on the rough stuff. If you fatigue muscles on a flat stretch, don't worry, the curved and wavy stuff up ahead will shake them loose.

On a perfectly flat cement path, however, the chance of an overuse injury goes up infinitely because you work your feet and legs in the exact same way, stride after stride, mile after mile. This is also why, even when you're shod, faster marathon times are often run on courses that are not perfectly flat. It keeps the feet and legs fresher, letting a greater number of muscles participate in the work.

Last challenge of the smooth surface. As you get faster and your soles harden, you'll find yourself sliding around a bunch. Get fast enough, and even with great form, your feet feel as if they're sliding on ice. Now this can be super for form and stability work, and for trying to get your smoothest stride ever. However, it's also a tough way to scuff off your pads without realizing it. Our feet are stimulated by pressure, not by sliding. Run cement paths day after day, and you'll likely sandpaper away all of your hard-earned gains.

◐°°°₀ FOOT NOTE

Road Best Traveled Less

Chip and seal roads are a cost-effective solution to pavement. These types of roads keep the windshield repair shops in business. Take one old road, add a good layer of hot, sticky oil, then throw down a layer of small sharp rocks. Count on pressure from passing cars, and voila, you have a "new" road, flying rocks, cracked windshields, and an overabundance of small, protruding rocks that could be a new way to think about reflexology if you run on them.

Asphalt or paved bike and running paths

These paths tend to be far kinder and more forgiving than the smooth cement ones. Yes, they're not quite as smooth, and therefore a bit more challenging if you're just getting into the game. However, once your feet toughen up a bit, chances are you'll come to like these surfaces. Asphalt is a combination of steam-rolled rocks and oil, and that combination adds far more spring to your step. The oil acts as a rubbery surface, making the ground softer and more forgiving. Additionally, it's not pancake flat. There are always imperfections and undulations in the pavement on asphalt. This helps keep your feet and legs fresh and helps prevent overuse injuries.

Like chip and seal, often the asphalt's not as smooth as we'd like. I've seen many park paths and bike paths with notably sharp pavement. While cement wears away your feet faster than asphalt, because asphalt is coarser, it can create blisters faster. This sharpness isn't easy in the beginning, and for quite a while may slow you down.

Asphalt also heats up fast. So you'll have to watch yourself in the summer, particularly in southern climes and at high altitude. The pavement's not just hot to the touch, but could even have patches of melted asphalt or rubberlike crack fillings that have turned to hot oily goop. Build up slowly to the hot stuff, then enjoy. (Personally, after my feet grow accustomed to the heat, I think hot pavement feels like a great, long, foot massage.)

Compared to cement, asphalt cools and heats much more quickly. In the winter, this means asphalt is better to run on in the daytime and more challenging at night. It'll warm up quickly with the sun, then shed heat quickly at night. So, after dark, head for the cement.

Hot goopy tar balls

I cannot recommend running on newly paved blacktop. They turn your feet black and are a potential hazard to your health, at least after prolonged exposure. Additionally, the fumes from newly paved roads are a known carcinogen. Prolonged exposure is not recommended. However, if it's not too hot, you might find the texture or the way it coats your foot quite enjoyable, at least for a step or two.

If it's not packed down well, you could find yourself picking up a bunch of tar and loose rocks with your feet, and those hurt! Also, be careful if you transition from the fresh asphalt to the dirt. Chances are you'll be gluing rocks into the pads of your feet. Last, don't do this too close to home, or you'll track it in with you, and onto your floors.

Older asphalt roads tend to be much coarser than newer ones, meaning you'll fatigue, soften, or even tenderize your feet faster than on the smooth stuff. They're also more likely to give you blisters faster than smooth surfaces. Watch for sharp angles and major cracks in the road that can catch or trip up your feet. Also watch for seams on the roads and the paths. They trip you up, particularly once you're fatigued.

Native American lore has it that an oil-like mixture was often applied to the bottoms of their feet to harden their skin once stripped bare of their winter moccasins. The oil in pavement may have such an effect of stimulating pad growth and tempering the feet; I just can't say that it's too healthy and can't be very natural.

Pockmarked sidewalks

Old, chewed-up, pockmarked sidewalks (and occasionally sloppy new sidewalks) are a hallmark of the East Coast life. It's as if someone took a chisel or jackhammer to the surface but forgot to finish the job. They're hard cement, but far from smooth, and quick to chew up your feet. I'd call these challenging and un-fun, even if you have tough, strong feet. They're just far too unpredictable.

It's hard to get into a rhythm or find your groove on these sidewalks, and you often find yourself clipping along and then sailing into a rough patch. Either that, or you never get going at all. If you have to run on these, jog lightly, particularly if they're even slightly wet. Better yet, avoid these minefields altogether if possible.

New England roads

Whether you live in the Northeast, or anywhere else that's truly pedestrian unfriendly and doesn't have sidewalks or shoulders on the roads, be careful. Of course we all understand the dangers of running with traffic and likely know to run on the left rather than right side of the road (so you can see what's coming and get out of harm's way or dive out of harm's way if necessary).

But these roads have an added dimension of danger: road debris. These old roads are often littered with glass, broken plastic, or even sharp wires from wornout retreaded truck tires on the sides of the roads. Run here, even with thickened pads, and you're asking for trouble. Best to find someplace else to run such as a local park, a nature preserve, or head for the local track if you're out of other options.

Tracks

There are three main types of tracks: cinder, paved, and rubber coated—each with its own unique challenges.

Cinder Tracks: Cinder's soft and can be a lot of fun (particularly if it's slightly moist), but you can slide around quite a bit. Also, depending on the coarseness, you can wear your feet down pretty good. However, Zola Budd (South African phenom and former world record holder in the 5K) was often photographed training barefoot on cinder tracks. Perhaps that's all they had for her to run on, but it served her feet well.

Paved Tracks: These tracks have all the challenges of pavement, yet with an added bonus—turns. Pavement's springier than cement, but far from forgiving when you're turning fast. It can chew up the sides of your feet quickly and put additional stress and strain on ligaments and tendons if you're not ready.

Rubber-Coated Tracks: These are fun and springy, but give you less feedback for your feet. It's hard to keep from striking hard, and as with all tracks, the perfectly flat surface makes it even easier to have an overuse injury. All tracks are bad for this because of the repetitive motion on the flats, but rubberized tracks are notorious, because you lack proper feedback for your feet.

If the rubber's new, it's likely quite coarse—perfect for traction, particularly in shoes, but also quick to burn away your padding, particularly on the tips of your outside toes. Watch for this, and if you sense or smell your feet burning, call it quits or throw on your shoes. Many a barefoot runner has been known to tape their toes to prevent friction from these surfaces. Personally, I've been known to apply a bit of Gorilla Glue SuperGlue or QuikCallus for track workouts. While the glue is not great for the feet, it wears off quickly on the track, and I'd rather wear off the glue than my skin or toes.

One last challenge with rubberized surfaces. Over the years, the thousands of runners who come through tend to wear grooves, patterns, or even make smooth the rubberized surfaces. At speed this makes you feel as if you're running on ice and can wear your feet down quickly (not to mention radically change your form). Watch for this and try to avoid grooved patterns and smooth spots. If unavoidable, watch your feet carefully, and be prepared to call it a day.

Whatever track you end up running on, alternate directions 50-50—or run 50 percent of your laps one direction, and 50 percent of your laps the other. This is exceptionally important, as the tight turns, particularly on the inner laps, put significant strain on your stabilizer muscles and all of the joints of your feet. If you run continuously in one direction lap after lap, or workout after workout, you're inviting a substantial overuse injury, and perhaps even a stress fracture.

When you think barefoot and track, think every third day. But no matter what surface, if you spend time at the track, plan on letting your pads recover for at least two days before hitting it again. First, you need the recovery from your speed workout. Second, no matter the surface, you've likely fatigued your pads and tired your muscles, ligaments, and tendons.

Dirt roads

Ahhh, the joy of getting *off* the hard stuff and onto something more natural—or at least *slightly* more natural. If you can find a good dirt road, you've found a friend for life. They're softer than pavement, have more natural undulations (which help prevent overuse injuries), and they help build pads.

Of course, there are different types of dirt and consistencies, but that's half the fun. Some are cement hard, others as soft as a beach. Some are sun-baked and cracked in the summer; others have dry, sharp angulations from muddy vehicles and footprints that dry incredibly hard. Still others become washboard-like from vehicles. The most challenging dirt roads are gravel filled.

All dirt roads help promote pad development. Watch for ice hidden in the dirt in the winter, and for sharp dried mud and clay and potentially thorns (in the Southwest)

in the summer. This dried mud can be the best at strengthening and toughening your entire foot, not just the parts that typically hit the ground. However, this also means you have to start light, as the skin and muscles around your arch and soft spots of the foot won't be ready for this. Do too much too quickly and you'll not only scuff up the bottom of your feet, but spectacularly bruise them as well.

Packed mud on dirt roads is also a fantastically fast surface. If there's any moisture, they tend to be grippy enough so as not to prematurely wear down your feet, but they help you zip along at incredible speeds. I think it's my favorite surface for going fast. I also love running a good washboard road and timing my strides to land on the peaks, almost hopping over the troughs.

I recommend trying out different dirt roads. Some you'll love, others you'll avoid. Just start into them slowly, then watch your feet grow naturally strong.

Gravel roads

Love 'em or leave 'em. Gravel's great for building your feet. Perhaps man was never meant to run on gravel. Although we can adapt to anything, gravel roads are a pain to get into. The rock on them isn't natural. It's chewed-up granite, sharpened at funny angles. These rocks don't move when you hit them, but stick straight up underfoot. There's no give, and did I mention? They're sharp.

Yet there's almost no better surface (except perhaps jagged dried mud) for building your pads and foot strength fast. Just start incredibly slowly. Consider walking 100 yards of it your first try, then call it quits. From there, build up gradually, venturing just a bit farther and slightly faster. What I love the most about gravel roads is that if you can master them, you can run on just about anything.

City sidewalks

Oddly enough, New York City's sidewalks are among my favorite running surfaces ever. They're incredibly smooth, worn down by millions of feet trodding along year after year; and they're not too hard. Perhaps best of all, the curbs tend to be smooth metal surfaces. This means you can run on sidewalks, dart onto the edge of the roads (be careful), leap onto a curb, back up, then down right again. It's almost like skateboarding, darting in and out, leaping small obstacles, and running your smoothest, fastest surface ever. While I'm a nature guy all the way, running Times Square or through the city can be a ton of fun (just make sure to wash your feet afterward; city streets are far dirtier than dirt itself).

◉°°₀ FOOT NOTE: Road Camber

Road camber is that slight pitch on the side of a road, path, or even single-track trail. Typically built for drainage, one side of the road or path is banked higher than the other, which can put undue strain on one leg, or even one ligament or tendon of a foot or leg, causing serious overuse injuries over time. But when you feel the ground, and land on your forefoot, you can easily compensate for camber.

I still try to avoid running on a cambered surface, but if it's unavoidable, I minimize the negative effects by going out on camber in one direction (let's say leaning to the left) and returning in the reverse or, if possible, alternating by switching sides back and forth. In this way, I balance out the work my muscles have had to do.

This type of adusting can't be done in shoes, because the body can't tell what's going on, underneath. It's only when you take the gloves off, so to speak, and feel what's beneath you that the body begins to wake up, to sense, to make changes and take action. And that's where the real fun and adaptation take place.

Hitting the Trails

When it comes to barefoot running, trails are what we were born to run on.

From a reflexology point of view, nothing stimulates your feet, and thereby everything in your entire body, than running on trails. You'll touch and stimulate each and every nerve ending of your foot, helping reduce blood pressure, relax your mind, and improve your overall health.

There are an unlimited number of types of trails, each with its own unique characteristics, traits, and challenges. One mile you're running on the soft stuff, the next dried sharp clay, the next bounding over rocks. This can be quite enjoyable. It keeps things from getting boring, gives your feet (and mind) a great workout, and keeps you from becoming fatigued.

Muddy trails

These are delightful to the feet. Now I'm a strong believer in protecting the environment and keeping bikes and shoes off the mud, but if you're out in the mud, it feels great. Perhaps I'm being a hypocrite, but there's something far more natural and less damaging about running barefoot through the mud. You leave far less of a footprint (pun intended) and find something strange; you do have traction. Our feet grip far better than shoes in the mud. We dig in with our toes, and if we stay on our forefeet, we keep from sliding around.

Just make sure, if you run in the mud, you're not damaging or destroying the trails. Mud's fun, but if there's a good chance of erosion, steer clear.

A great benefit of mud? Not only does it feel soothing, but it protects your feet. If the mud cakes on, you've created a natural shoe. Going from muddy conditions to rocky conditions is a blast; the mud protects your feet and lets you safely run the jagged stuff. Of course, if the mud's still wet and you hit the dirt, you may pick up more than you bargained for—like rocks sticking to your feet.

I love starting a barefoot run by running in, jumping in, or stepping in a mud puddle to protect and moisturize without softening the bottom of my feet.

Icy muddy trails

Although running in the mud feels great, and can be good for you too, you want to be careful if the mud is part of a snow melt/thaw. If so, the ground may be below freezing, the mud at 32 degrees, and wet snow and puddles may abound. If that's the case, even winterized feet may get cold, fast. The high moisture content along with the mud cools feet quickly, then encases them in cold cement. Even if you're a conditioned snow runner, be wary or avoid these conditions.

If you do decide to shed your shoes, realize you're committed. If your feet get too cold, there's no warming them up on the trail; the encased mud will keep your feet cold, and there's little chance of stuffing the mud balls (or your clown feet) back into your shoes. Instead, you're gonna have to ride it out, or sprint it out. It's also difficult to grab with your toes when they're getting cold in mud and ice and fairly encased, which affects traction and squashes your arches.

If you've truly made friends with the snow, these conditions may still be fine. Just make sure you don't destroy the trail while having fun and get your feet clean of mud before you enter your car. Why? Because even with your car heater blasting, the mud will continue to cool off your feet during your drive or at least prevent them from warming up. Before you get back in your car, I recommend jogging on the roads if at all possible to warm up your feet and clean off the mud.

Rocky trails

This is head's-up running at its finest. Make sure to run with your eyes scanning the horizon, everywhere from 6 to 8 feet in front of you and beyond. Over time, you'll learn to see what's coming ahead and what's beneath your feet simultaneously. This is important because you'll find yourself bounding from rock to rock in rhythm with the trail. Always focus on what's ahead and never stride past your field of vision.

If you can't see where your feet are falling, slow down until your mind catches up. It's a muscle too and will learn to coordinate your feet and the rocks so you know where to step and land with accuracy.

Running rocks can be a meditative experience. There's something stimulating, yet relaxing about running the rocks. It's incredibly powerful for quieting the mind. Why? Because when the mind's completely focused on picking your steps, there's no room for stray thoughts to enter.

Things to watch for: loose rocks, gravel, and big rocks with lips.

Hitting gravel on the trails can be quite a surprise, particularly when you're bounding through the rocks. Do your best to instantly lower the landing gear, get your arms down, and lower that center of gravity.

Tall rocks and rocks with overhangs are famous for skinning the tops of your toes. At these times you'll wish you had hair on the back of your feet. But not to worry, without scarring, the skin quickly grows back stronger, making them far more scuff-resistant the next time around. Additionally, hitting rocks or scuffing your feet helps build new eyes in your feet, helping your mind and feet become more pro-active. With practice, you'll know exactly where to place the feet and hit your mark with the accuracy of an Olympic archer.

If you can't hop from rock to rock, then look for smooth surfaces on which to land. If you can't find them, you'll find your feet landing at funny angles at strange protruding surfaces. This is great for strengthening your feet and building your pads. Just make sure to stop once you've fatigued your feet. After the feet tire, you're incredibly susceptible tripping on such uneven surfaces. At times like these, consider putting on your shoes and walking your way back out of there.

Mountain climbs

Like mountains? Love to be vertical? Then you may become hooked on barefoot mountain runs. It's on the vertical where you find out what your toes were meant to do. Your feet become like a second set of hands, able to grab and pull you up on even the steepest of terrain.

With strong bare feet, you'll be able to run stuff you'd never consider with shoes, and with far greater ease and balance. However, you not only want to start slow with short distances on the steep stuff, but consider wearing your shoes for the downhill. Many trail runners, myself included, got into mountain climbs this way. It lets us work and fatigue our feet on the uphill, and then when they're tired, we turn around, slip on our shoes, and slowly make our way back home.

Mountain runs are incredible at building up your feet. Once you've accomplished them, bask in the glory of your effort. You've done something special.

The Ins and Outs of Trail Running

There's a strange puddle out in the middle of nowhere on a trail I frequent. It looks as if it's coated with oil, year-round. How a puddle remains in sub-zero temperatures I'm just not sure, and I'm quite wary, too. I have no idea what lurks beneath that puddle, but I have to assume it's nothing good.

Running in mud can be a lot of fun, but if there are pools of water that don't drain, particularly if you're in a warm climate, beware. While the risk of worms and parasites is quite low in this country, festering puddles are fair breeding grounds for these wee-beasties.

Best advice, if you're running in an unsanitary place (such as many third-world countries) or a place where water stagnates, stay out of the mud and free-standing water. And if you still play in the mud, don't stop for long periods of time. It's said that the creepy crawlers truly crawl onto your feet (you'll often feel them) when you stop. Keep a move on.

ⓞ°°°。 FOOT NOTE

Always bring your shoes to mountains; you never know what's going to happen—from weather, terrain, or even injury—even just a few miles from home. Trek in, and you'll have to trek out, no matter what. So bring shoes that will get you out. Better safe than sorry.

Barefoot hiking

Trail hiking, particular on hills, is the perfect way to build into barefoot running. It helps strengthen the feet, give them greater flexibility, build stronger skin, and perhaps above all else, gets you out into nature with the earth beneath your feet, faster and sooner than you ever could by running.

While barefoot hiking promotes better running, it's an ideal activity unto itself.

Exercise: Pick Your Path

Look for a trail nearby that's not too rocky to begin with. Often these are mountain bike trails, because the bikes tend to chew up and soften the dirt and spit the rocks out to the sides. Go exploring, even with your shoes on, to find the best trails to begin.

Try this: When you head out for your first adventure, carry your shoes with you as hand weights or put them in a lightweight pack. Don't set a goal of getting to the top of a mountain or hill, or going a certain distance. Just go out and gently walk the trail. Try to stand as tall as you can, keep the core tight, your belly button snapped to your spine, and that string pulling you to the sky.

Start with short distances, perhaps walking for 10 to 20 minutes, then put the shoes on and turn around.

If you've been doing this for weeks, gradually increase the time on rocks and more technical terrain. Consider adding 5 to 10 minutes each time you go out.

What do you do when you're out there? Just take your time and have fun. Everything's opposite on the trails from what you'd imagine. Large rocks (formerly the scariest things on the trail) become great stepping stones and platforms. Meanwhile, the easiest, most worn part of the trail may be the most difficult, lined with little pebbles. Pick your path carefully, but try not to look at the ground. Instead look at an imaginary horizon in front of you, and let your gaze reach to the ground.

Don't worry about your speed or destination, just have fun, and connect with the earth, one bare foot at a time.

Ups and Downs of Hills

Uphills help strengthen your feet and get you into barefoot running. Even before you run, you can begin walking barefoot up a neighborhood hill, then jog on down in your shoes. Walk slightly on your toes to help strengthen things fast and grab with your toes. The uphill motion puts lots of pressure on your skin, which greatly helps build your pads. The motion also helps keep you on your toes and off your arches.

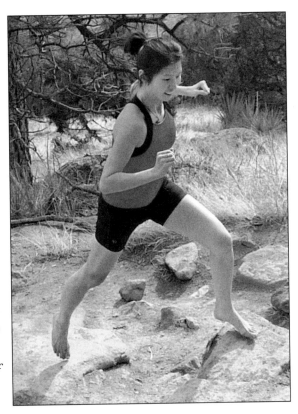

Note how Jessica bounds from forefoot to forefoot, all while staying tall. Never bend forward, but let that string pull you to the sky. Stay light and you'll see yourself fly up even the steepest terrain.

Uphill running is a strength trainer and foot conditioner as well. It helps you get on your toes with minimal impact. However, start slowly as your ankles and stabilizing muscles may be quite weak, and your dorsiflexors on your toes (muscles that pull your toes up) are likely weak if not dormant. When you run up hills, your dorsiflexors help to keep your toes up to prevent stubbing them. This action quickly becomes natural, particularly if you accidentally stub one or two. However, these muscles and the associated ligaments are likely atrophied if you've been shod your entire life.

Although you can start walking up hills almost right away, I recommend building feet for two months before running uphill. Then do it every second or third workout, to give yourself plenty of time to recover.

Over time, the hills will help you progress quickly and get your heart and lungs working too. Running downhills barefoot is far more intense and stressful on the foot than running uphills. As with walking, start by throwing on shoes for the downhill and taking things ridiculously slow.

Uphill trail running is another fantastic workout. I'd recommend starting by walking uphill barefoot, then walking down in shoes. Do this once a week for about a month before you try jogging the uphills. Always bring your shoes with you, and until you're confident, slip on your shoes and walk the downhills.

The difficulty of every surface is exaggerated by uphills. Even if you're used to the rocks on the flats, they'll be more challenging on the uphills. The great news is, in the beginning, you can get as good a workout hiking up the hills as running on the roads. So don't worry about taking it slow—be the tortoise and have fun with it.

⦿°°°₀ FOOT NOTE

You can lean into the uphill slightly to let gravity work for you, instead of against you; however, never pivot at the hips and bend forward into the uphill. This robs you of all your power and puts tremendous stress and strain on your shins, ankles, hamstrings, and knees. You want to keep yourself tall even or especially on the uphills and let the silver string pull you toward the sky.

What goes up . . .

A common question at clinics and talks is whether you can stay on your toes when running downhill barefoot. People have often been taught that to run a downhill you want to relax and dig in with your heels, letting your legs slow you down. However, shod or not, this is actually a dangerous way to drive force up through your joints and back and hurt yourself badly over time.

The best technique for downhills, whether on road or trail, is to stand tall, keep your arms up, and lean back slightly, letting gravity slow you down. Keep your core tight, and never bend forward at the waist. You want to stay on your toes, no matter what, because it helps absorb the shock, and keeps you better balanced. You'll find on the trails, whether downhill or not, the times you slip and slide are when you're on your heels. When you keep pressure on your toes, you help maintain traction. (This technique takes time to master. Introduce time barefoot on downhills slowly. Even consider walking 100 yards, then jogging 100 yards, then repeating.)

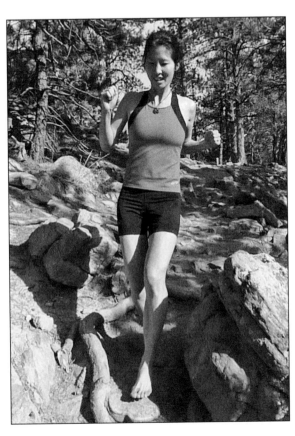

While running downhill, always look ahead and stand tall. Keep your arms up, never lean for- ward, and stay on your toes to remain agile and nimble (so you can react fast). Then smile!

The secret to great downhills is leg speed. Work to pick your legs back up fast and carry them through fast. Picture your legs moving as if you were pedaling a unicycle. Keeping your strides short but fast helps you fly down hills and even mountains with little or no impact at all. (Practice the Butt Kick drill explained in an earlier chapter to help with leg turnover for downhills.)

Downhills are unique in running. They require you to decelerate with each step. Fortunately, if you're keeping your strides short, there's little impact or force on your joints; however, your muscles are getting the workout of a lifetime. This is because downhills require your muscles to lengthen as they contract, rather than shorten. This is called an eccentric muscle contraction.

Eccentric muscle contractions are fantastic for building muscle control and strength. It's the same concept as lowering the muscle slowly in weightlifting but far more explosive. If you've heard of plyometrics, a concept made famous by Soviet athletes during the Cold War, Soviet athletes were found jumping over boxes and even off brick walls 11 feet high—a determining factor as to whether someone was allowed in the track and field program or not. Plyometrics help athletes by forcing the muscles to handle repetitive eccentric contractions. These contractions build muscle incredibly fast, but also can tear the heck out of them and create instant tendonitis.

Every step you take on a downhill is an eccentric muscle contraction. This is more than double the force the muscle has to do on the flats and a reason it's particularly important to get into downhills slowly. With eccentric muscle contractions on downhills rest assured, you're going to have DOMS (delayed onset muscle soreness) after your first few downhill workouts. So it's essential you only do one downhill workout a week for the first few months you're running hills.

Over time your body adapts, and your legs become incredibly fast and strong even for the flats. Then you can run downhills far more often and without the need for a lengthy recovery. But until that point, take it easy on the downhills, emphasize extra recovery, and take the day off after each and every downhill run.

◉°°°₀ FOOT NOTE

Begin with running a few hundred yards downhill your first time, then add another 100 to 200 yards each additional time. This will help keep you from tearing things apart as you break your legs in. Remember, running on the flats subjects your body to two and a half times the impact of your body weight with each and every step. On downhills you can easily double this number or more, which is why it's so essential to start slowly and let patience be your guide.

Running downhill on the trails is just like running downhill on the road, but with an added degree or two of difficulty. You're likely running downhill on loose and uneven surfaces, all the while having to hop over seen and unseen obstacles.

Downhill running on trails is truly an eye-opening, head's-up, challenging experience at first, and not for the faint of heart. It requires months of training on basic trails and uphills before you're ready. And then, when the time comes, should be done for a few hundred yards to begin with at most. After that point your legs will be wobbly and unstable. Should you continue, you're likely in for a fall.

When you begin, try to find a trail that doesn't have a lot of golf-ball-sized rocks or smaller. These are the hardest to handle at first and cause the most pain. You're looking for your feet to gain eyes, so they can find their own foot placement on the downhills. Meanwhile, look ahead and pick the exact spots for your landings.

It takes time for your nervous system to adapt to the downhills and properly control your feet, legs, and balance. Leg speed, balance, and grace only come after great repetition. Repetition builds muscle memory—an adaptation by your nervous system to do something smoothly, efficiently, and automatically.

Until your muscles and mind work as one on downhills, you're likely to feel awkward, far from light, and quickly imbalanced or fatigued. Not to worry, our minds will figure this out, and over time help us to dance on the downhills.

Cross the Bridge When You Come to It

If you run on city paths, or near the coast, you'll likely have to cross your fair share of bridges. They're often nothing to worry about, but can understandably be intimidating to beginners.

There are only two types of bridges you have to watch for: metal-grated bridges and old wooden bridges typically filled with splinters. If you run on metal grates, run particularly slowly and make sure you lower your landing gear to increase your surface area and keep from bouncing. Try a step or two precariously. You may find you have to walk the bridge—or even temporarily put on your shoes.

The best way to break into metal bridge walks is by spending time barefoot on escalators or moving walkways that you find in airports. They'll strengthen your feet and provide the same kind of force as the metal-grated bridge, yet without nearly the edge on them.

As for wooden bridges, though I've never gotten a splinter from one, no matter how worn the bridge is, I'm still always wary. I try to avoid them if I can, and if not, I think light and try to float my way across the bridge. I'll try to keep myself pointed forward too. The less I try to turn and pivot on the old wood, the less chance I'll pick up something undesirable.

Night Running

Did you know your feet have eyes? Running barefoot, we can sense the terrain in front of us and adjust on the fly, *especially* in the dark. My favorite barefoot runs are out on trails in total darkness.

You would think that'd be the perfect time of day to kill yourself; but if you run without ego, and succumb to the trail, if you simply *allow* the trail to come your way, then you can almost do no harm.

Many of our students have reported the easiest time of day to run is after dark. They experience no longer stepping on small stones, pebbles, or even branches, as if all obstacles magically disappear. Once our true eyesight diminishes, we're more likely to relax and let go, rather than staying tense and fighting the terrain. Our feet and subconscious take over and sense the trail for us. Running light and on the forefoot too gives our feet a chance to negotiate whatever comes our way. Forefoot landing with the foot out allows extra time for the feet to find their path. We're not locked as we are in a shoe, but free for the feet to pick and choose their way.

Our minds are incredibly fast, our nervous systems even faster. We simply need to get out of our way, get out of thought, and perhaps even get out of sight (something our modern society, culture, and world is madly obsessed about in a very unbalanced way). When our eyesight can't serve us, or like a blind man whose sense of hearing becomes talk of legend, our other senses kick in. If we let these senses take over, then our super-sensitive feet have the time and the knowledge to guide us down the trail.

Ironically, the more you run in the dark, the better your night vision becomes too. This heightened sense of awareness helps you fly through the night and guides you on your way.

Exercises: Out of Sight, In Our Mind

Try this: Once you're comfortable running barefoot—after perhaps a few months—try going for a night run on a dimly lit trail or bike path for a mile or two. Start someplace safe, where you're not likely to get mugged, or eaten by a bear or big cat, but don't turn on that headlight.

Instead, let your body feel its way along the trail. In the daytime, you have a tendency to hunt and peck for every rock along the trail, overly concerned you'll hit them, and because of this, when you do, you're tense and they hurt. But at night you can't look for the tiny pebbles. All you can do is relax into them, and that's where the fun begins. Something strange happens when you hit the pebbles you can't see at night. They don't hurt nearly as much, or you may not even feel them at all because you've relaxed your body and your feet and just flow or give into the rocks, rather than tense up and fight them.

Try this: Learn to see without eyes: Find your way blindfolded. This may seem crazy at first, but it's practiced by many Native American tribes as well as the Lung-Gom-Pa and other running and spiritual people around the world.

Start with walking or jogging slowly an incredibly simple trail, then work your way into more complex, rocky terrain. While it's tempting to do this with a partner, you'll likely use them too much as a crutch. Instead go someplace you know is safe, where there are no steep dropoffs, or other major obstacles to contend with, and start with 100 feet or less at a time. Then simply focus on your breath, breathing slow, deep, and controlled, and let your feet do the walking.

I was once stuck miles from anywhere, deep in the woods after dark, with my two dogs, Pumpkin and Sawa. I was wearing my Asics Piranha, a 4.2-ounce racing flat with no support and superb ground feel for a running shoe, while dancing through the woods on my toes. But when it got dark, it got really dark. No moon above, I was buried in the woods.

I expected to trip, stumble, and fall with every footstep, particularly because I didn't want to slow down as I felt the need to get home. But running on my forefeet, something strange happened. I was running light, almost tapping the ground with my toes. And I never tripped, not once. By landing on my toes, my feet were able to feel and find the ground, stabilizing me with each step.

It was a magical run home—6 to 8 miles of total bliss in the darkness. With only stars to guide our way, and the ground beneath our feet, we were in silence, and in heaven. It was incredibly peaceful, and strangely enough, there were no signs of fatigue when we got to the car.

Perhaps that's why I like running at night best. You connect with the world around you, become one with the trails, and you let your other senses guide you. Your eyes no longer are your strongest sense, but play a supporting role. Instead you feel your way, guided by the ground, silence, and intuition.

Get out of the city, off the beaten path, and don't be afraid to explore. If you start slowly, your body can handle much more than you ever gave it credit for. It can overcome and adapt to incredible conditions: gravel trails, sloppy mud paths, endless hills, cold metal bridges, and dark of night. Not only that, but feeling the ground—your connection with nature—and the sense of accomplishment you'll gain will have you grinning from ear to ear as you run. So be a child again, explore, see things anew, and have fun!

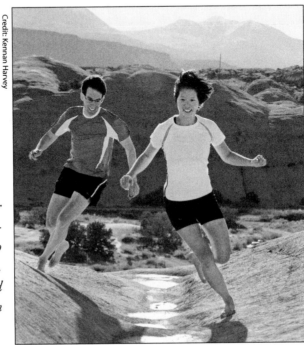

Credit: Kennan Harvey

You gain a childlike awe for the world and agility you never knew you had once you go barefoot and touch the earth. It's pure joy as Jessica and Michael skip on slickrock in Moab, Utah.

12

Overcoming the Agony of the Feet

I can't be funny if my feet don't feel right.
—Billy Crystal

Whether you're struggling with a long-term injury, just getting into barefoot running, or are years into the game, understanding injuries and their potential causes and solutions can help you get and stay healthy—and recover in the event of an injury. In this chapter we'll look at many of the common challenges facing runners, shod and unshod. Expect to toss more than a few myths and common misconceptions about barefoot running by the wayside.

People often ask, don't you worry about getting injured when running barefoot? To them I respond, "The greater risk is getting injured in a shoe. So what have I got to lose?" In a shoe or out, accidents sometimes happen. We run too far, we do too much, or we twist an ankle or trip.

At the same time, we've all heard the warnings: Barefoot running is hazardous to your health. Local doctors and podiatrists warn in print and TV, the barefoot running trend will get you hurt. But are they right?

Yes. If you've been in shoes and don't transition slowly to barefoot running, it's almost inevitable you'll tear yourself apart and find yourself quickly sidelined with tendonitis, stress fractures, or other problems.

But these injuries are avoidable. Follow these simple rules of the road and you're well on your way.

Top 10 Rules of the Road for a Healthy Transition to Barefoot Running

1. **Go Slow.** Consider starting with 100 to 200 yards and then building with 100 additional yards every other day.

2. **Let Your Skin Be Your Guide.** Going barefoot to begin, even if you love your Vibram FiveFingers, helps you feel the ground, gain awareness, wake up the feet (circulation, nerves, skin, and more) and learn to run light.

3. **Build Foot Strength.** Don't just go out and run. Work on foot-strengthening exercises in between runs.

4. **Focus on Form.** Running barefoot demands great form. Consult Chapter 5 on getting started.

5. **Leave the iPod and Ego Behind.** Running barefoot requires your attention and awareness when you begin. Don't worry, you can get back to your music and goals soon enough.

6. **Get Balanced.** Work on balance and symmetrical strength. Asymmetrical weaknesses are a huge cause of injuries, in and out of a shoe.

7. **Get Loose.** Commit to stretching in new ways, primarily with a foam roll or balls. Also consider massages or massage machines to help get and keep the blood flowing and get the muscles loose.

8. **Get Aligned.** Mechanical misalignments, typically caused by asymmetrical strength, weaknesses, and tightness can pull, push, twist, and contort your body, forcing you to run misaligned, quickly creating overuse injuries.

9. **Go Bare.** This doesn't mean running barefoot all the time, but it means getting your feet out of shoes and (preferably) feeling uneven surfaces. You'll get the greatest workout in the world by forcing your body to constantly adjust and shift the micro-vasculature of the feet—in essence, bathing your feet in oxygen and nutrients for greater recovery, flexibility, and strength building.

10. **Learn to Rest.** No matter how diligent you are, if you don't take time off to recover, you'll tear yourself apart. Begin barefoot running with no more than every-other-day sessions for the first 3 months. If you feel a tweak, head for home, rest between workouts, and don't head out when you're sore.

Although there's no way to cover every conceivable injury or pain (that's what entire professions are for), I'll do my best to cover the basics. A caveat here, when in doubt, always see a doctor (preferably a barefoot friendly one). I am not a doctor, nor do I play one on TV. And the lawyers urge me to tell you that you should use caution when it comes to your health. Advice given here is not professional medical advice.

That said, here's what works best for me and other barefoot runners (and maybe for you too).

First, the First Aid

Cuts

The most common worry in the beginning classes I teach is getting cut by broken glass, sharp rocks, and other jagged objects. The truth is that serious cuts are among the least common injuries suffered by barefoot runners. Once you're aware of your surroundings and have toughened up your feet, you'll avoid most sharp objects and be relatively shielded from the rest.

If you do suffer a serious cut, though, the first thing to do is stop running. Consider your session done for the day, and your only job is to attend to the injury. If the cut is deep, do not seal it up until you've let the blood push out the dirt, bacteria, and other sources of infection. Let the wound air out until it's clean.

If it's a deep puncture wound, consider seeking medical help. You may need your doctor to completely clean it out and also to give you a tetanus booster shot to prevent infection (update tetanus every 10 years). But if you can't remember when you had a shot and it's been more than 5 years, you're likely to get a booster anyway.

Once you've cleaned the wound as best you can on the spot with clean water, put on your shoes (assuming you brought them along as hand weights); get home; clean the wound thoroughly with hydrogen peroxide, Betadine, or some other sanitizing solution. If it's small, let it breathe. If not, cover the cut up with a bandage or a product such as Spenco's 2nd Skin. Before you go out again, use products such as 3M's Nexcare or QuikCallus to seal and protect the cut. Don't even think of running barefoot unless the cut is sealed or protected. Never go out with an open wound.

And don't think for an instant about running again until the wound is fully healed.

Cracks

One key to healthy feet is keeping the skin from cracking. Drying out the skin may help toughen things up, but if you're constantly fighting crack after crack, you're not doing yourself much good. Personally, I've struggled with keeping the skin on my big toes and heels from cracking. I've tried and had some success with the following:

- Aloe

- Climb On!

- Coconut oil

- Sesame seed oil

- Vaseline (petroleum jelly)

- Shea butter

- Joshua's Tree Cycling Salve

All of these work best if you're dealing with a new crack. However, if the crack is further along in development, consider sealing it with 3M's Nexcare or QuikCallus to protect and aid in recovery.

Apparently, cracked skin is a common phenomenon with bare feet. According to Hendrick Maako, a marathoner who grew up running barefoot in South Africa, runners used Vaseline to keep their feet moisturized and prevent cracking. He said, "You could always tell if someone used Vaseline on their feet. You could see their feet shining a mile away!"

I recommend keeping your feet dry and clean, bathing and showering frequently, and applying salves, oil, creams, or petroleum jelly at night, particularly on any trouble spots to keep the skin from cracking. Various products and concoctions seem to work better than others, and all work in their own way. The trick is finding a balance between keeping the skin moist enough that it doesn't crack, and dry enough that it's not too soft to wear away when you run. Do not use straight moisturizers, which destroy the pads you've worked so hard to gain. You want to prevent cracks without softening the skin.

Infections

Another fear of beginners is that they'll step in something nasty and get an infection. To reduce the odds, try this:

- Run aware so you don't step in anything bad. For example, in a park beware of dog deposits; and in the woods, keep an eye out for other animal droppings. Stay away from stagnating pools of water (especially in hot, moist climates). And avoid unsanitary areas—or if you can't, stop running and put on your shoes until you're clear of them.

- Always keep a sanitizer such as hydrogen peroxide or Betadine, or a towel with soapy water, waiting by your door. You may have stepped in something disgusting without even realizing it. And even if you were running in a beautiful wooded area, you might have picked up unwanted passengers such as ticks. Rather than track the remnants of your day's adventures through your foyer, living room, and bedroom, make a habit of thoroughly examining and washing your feet and legs as soon as you arrive home.

- Keep your immunizations current and know when you get them. If you suffer a puncture wound, you'll be spared a tetanus shot if you clearly remember that you've already had one within the past 10 years.

The moment your feet feel raw, end your run. This rule actually applies across the board, but it's especially pertinent to ensuring your feet aren't susceptible to penetration. If your feet get soft, tender, or raw, you're liable to get cut.

Common Aches, Pains, and Injuries from the Bottom Up

Leg length discrepancies

Causes: Many people are born with an undiagnosed leg length discrepancy—one leg is longer than the other. If you were never in shoes, this would never be a problem because the body would feel the ground and find a way to get balance. However, in a shoe, that becomes darn near impossible. According to an article published in *Podiatry Today*, "Leg length asymmetries appear to be the third most common cause of running injuries and occur in 60 to 90 percent of the population." While most leg length discrepancies are small, some may be more than a centimeter to an inch or greater due to traumatic injury.

Solution: Gradually work into getting balanced by feeling the ground through barefoot walking and running. See how using road camber can be helpful (you'll find this information in the chapter on exploring terrain).

Plantar fasciitis or pain on the bottom of the foot

Causes: A big sign you have plantar fasciitis is pain on the bottom of your feet or heels with your first few morning steps. (If you've ever wondered how to pronounce this painful condition, it's *planter fash-ee-eye-tis*.) Tendonitis and irritation on the bottom of the foot is a common problem caused by weak muscles and poor circulation on the bottom of the foot. Poor circulation comes from a trapped foot that's unable to feel the ground or move freely. And weak muscles are a common condition in a foot that's been inhibited in a shoe (and can't move like a spring) or where there's too much arch support digging into the foot.

Before you go barefoot, it's very common when the plantar fascia, or connective tissue on the bottom of the foot, is forced to do the supportive work of the weak and atrophied muscles of the foot. Since this tissue was never designed for such a job, it can quickly become inflamed.

Solution: Barefoot running can help strengthen the feet and chase your plantar fasciitis away. However, you have to start slowly (consider beginning with a 100-yard jog)

and never go barefoot if you're in acute pain. If you are weightlifting, go barefoot for a short time; then rest and use your supportive orthotics or shoes until your next workout. When I began barefoot running, I had plantar fasciitis and was told I had the world's flattest feet. Getting up on your forefoot and taking pressure off your midfoot when walking or running helps too.

The slow and gradual building up of my own foot muscles—and the creation of an arch where I virtually had none before—put the support work back on my muscles where it belonged, allowing the plantar fascia tissue to heal. Doing too much, too quickly, can make this condition worse.

Heel spurs

Causes: Unchecked plantar fasciitis, which continues to get worse, may often lead to heel spurs as well as heel striking, considered a leading culprit in the latest research (it's hypothesized that heel spurs develop to be a protective skeletal response to stress or microfractures to protect the heel from impact). These spurs are calcium deposits or bony scar tissue caused by excess pulling by the plantar fascia on its attachment to the heel. Unfortunately, it's incredibly painful. It's called a *spur* because it'll dig in, like the spurs on a cowboy's boots, with each and every step. This is to be avoided at all costs.

Solution: Going barefoot, even walking on the forefoot (and taking pressure off the plantar fascia and off of the arch), can help with heel spurs, as it's critical to get your feet strong and alleviate the tension on your plantar fascia. You'll want to begin slowly, ice regularly, and take your time. Bone doesn't change overnight, so realize that even after your feet have gotten strong, it could be many months or longer for recovery. Focus on strength and exercises that don't irritate your heel. Use support when you're not strengthening your feet. Physical therapy, massages to the area, ultrasound, acupuncture, and other scar-tissue reducing measures may be helpful in reducing the spur, once you've got the functional reason resolved.

◐°°°₀ FOOT NOTE

How to Ice Your Feet

Use ice to cool down your feet after a workout and to prevent inflammation (for faster recovery).

For injury, mild or severe, I like Mueller adjustable cold/hot pack wraps. You simply keep them in the freezer until you need them (they're reusable). Then strap the pack around your foot or leg with the Velcro wrap. Easy. Improvise with a bag of frozen peas and an Ace bandage. Prop your legs up the wall and rotate the ice packs on and off for 20 minutes at least several times.

For simply cooling down, use ice for 5 to 10 minutes after a workout unless it's really hot outside or it's been a long run. Then ice for 20 minutes on any and all sore joints too.

Pain on top of the foot or on top of the big toe

Causes: One of the most common challenges when transitioning into barefoot running. Typically it's tendonitis, though if early warning signs aren't heeded (sometimes there aren't many), tendonitis can foreshadow or quickly proceed into stress fractures of the metatarsals. Tendonitis can also be caused by feet that are rotated to the sides—typically a long-term condition caused by motion control, over-supportive shoes, or hip strength and flexibility imbalances. Also watch for small aches, pains, or fatigue that will cause you to change your stride—another common situation that causes this tendonitis to begin.

Both tendonitis and stress fractures have the same cause: too much, too fast, misalignment, or poor form. This is the most common injury when you transition, particularly in a minimalist shoe. The full freedom of movement and flexibility of the foot feels great, but can bite you quickly if you don't let your skin be your guide. Foot and toe pain can also be caused by running at an unnatural pace (too fast or too slow), running with a weighted pack without building up, or hopping into treadmill running too quickly. In short, if the muscles aren't ready, they'll pull on the tendons causing inflammation.

Solution: Back off, rest, ice after workouts, wear shoes that rest your feet (such as racing flats, which have a bit less flexibility), and work to stretch your toes and legs out (tightness throughout the legs and hips at this time can exacerbate the condition). Additionally, keep walking lightly every other day (or more) on uneven surfaces to keep up the blood flow in your feet to expedite healing. Tread lightly. The condition usually subsides within 2 to 4 weeks, though any tendonitis can last from 6 to 8 weeks. After you've healed, start slowly, focus on form, and let your skin guide you.

Bruised big toe

Causes: A common condition when you begin, it's the little rocks that tend to get your big toes, right on the outside edge.

Solution: Other than a bit of rest, there's not much you can do for them. The good news is the area will become stronger and more resistant in the future.

Toe fractures or impact fractures

Causes: Hitting your toes or forefoot into a rock when running unaware or in minimalist footwear where you don't quite feel the ground.

Solution: If you think you've fractured your toe or foot, see your doctor. Chances are you'll need 4 to 6 weeks of rest, unless it's your smallest toe. If it's your small toe, the medical professionals may tell you there's nothing you can do, so let pain be your guide. For either type of toe injury, work on running more aware, in or out of a shoe.

Bruised or bloodied nails

Causes: If you've hit a rock really hard, you may have damaged a nail or soft tissue beneath the nail.

Solution: If you're in severe pain or there's swelling under the toe, this is the time to see a doctor. Either way, you may have to wait it out, and there's a chance your nail will fall off. The doctor may relieve the pressure by drilling a small hole in your nail (don't try this at home).

Ingrown toenails

Causes: Ingrown toenails are a common condition among shod runners and, in particular, distance runners and ultra-runners. They're typically caused by a toe that's squashed in a shoe and pressed up against the side of the shoe. Without anywhere to go, the toenail grows into the toe rather than out.

As a former shod runner, I fought diligently to keep from needing to see a podiatrist for my ingrown nails, constantly performing "minor bathroom surgery" on my nails to keep them in check. I've known runners who've gone as far as to have their toenails surgically altered or even removed to prevent reoccurrence of this painful condition.

Solution: As a barefoot runner, the answer is simple. Simply get out of your shoes and your nails won't be squashed into the sides of your toes. Now you may need to see a podiatrist at first to clean things up to begin with, but out of shoes, the condition should take care of itself.

Out of shoes the chance of growing disgusting fungus and molds goes way down too, as there's no anaerobic (lack of oxygen) dark, dirty, place for them to grow.

Scraped skin on the feet

Causes: If you've scraped your feet against rocks, branches, or other surfaces, they'll likely get cut up, at least until the skin grows stronger.

Solution: Simply clean up the scrapes with an antiseptic and let them heal, preferably with good contact with the air. The skin in this area will grow back stronger than ever. Native American kick-stick racers used to kick their feet against trees to get the skin stronger. I can't recommend this, but the skin does grow stronger and more resistant in a short time. Never run barefoot with open wounds.

Bruised heels

Causes: Just like it sounds. Ouch!

Solution: Stop smacking your feet on the ground and let them heal.

Ankle strains and sprains

Causes: The number one acute injury in a shoe. Fortunately, it's far less of a problem when you're not wearing shoes and are closer to the ground and can feel the ground. It'd be very difficult (though never impossible) to twist an ankle under such circumstances.

Solution: If you've sprained or strained an ankle and are in a lot of pain or if it's changed color or bruised (particularly below the ankle), get to a doctor and make sure you haven't torn or broken anything. If they tell you it's a sprained ankle and will never fully heal or be 100 percent, they're operating in the old paradigm. They're right it will never heal 100 percent in a shoe, but out of a shoe, your foot will find a way to get additional blood flow to the area to strengthen it more than ever before. So even if you've been told you have permanently weak ankles, this can be changed.

Pain around and just above the ankles

Causes: Typically soreness or mild tendonitis is caused by weak stabilizing muscles and instability around the ankles. This is common if you start into barefoot running too quickly. It can also occur if you're wearing too heavy of a shoe and the muscles around and above the ankles aren't used to carrying the weight (something they were never designed to do in nature). This is also often a problem if you've been barefoot over the summer or using the most minimal of footwear, and then go to something heavier or more substantial for the winter.

Solution: Goes away quickly with rest. Use a foam roller to roll out your legs and reduce muscle tension, and work on barefoot walking rather than running for a few days. Consider massage or a strong foot massager to help increase blood flow. Then build back more slowly. Work on balance and stability exercises too. Once you're more stable, these problems should go away. If they're mild, ice after workouts, and never work out these muscles two days in a row. (If the problem's from heavy footwear, back off the big boots, rest, then try to find lighter solutions.)

Shin splints

Causes: Shin splints are an insidious problem. You rest, they feel better. You run again, the pain returns. Shin splints are caused by a rotational or sheering force along the front of your leg as your leg wants to go one way, and your shoe forces it another. No matter how much you rest, the pain returns as soon as you're back in your shoe.

Solution: Run barefoot and up on your toes. The less time in a shoe, the less the rotational force. Of course, rest and ice if it's just begun, and never start barefoot running if you're in acute pain. However, if you're starting into more minimal shoes and the pain's just started, hop out of your shoes and jog around a block or two. Chances are it'll take your shins out of spasm, relax tight muscles, and help strengthen and tone weakened ones. A bit of barefoot jogging after a run in shoes can help hit the reset button for your shins and other tweaks, aches, and pains.

Tight (or shredded) calves and Achilles tendonitis

Causes: This is the number one short-term problem when starting barefoot running or developing a forefoot stride. We were (intended) in nature to run barefoot, but if we've spent a lifetime in a shoe, our calves and Achilles are shortened and weak. Running barefoot or on your forefoot is like doing 50 to 100 calf raises and plyometric stretches each minute. Without preparation this action will quickly shred ill-prepared calves and Achilles.

Solution: If your calves or Achilles are sore, take time to let them rest before you go again, which may be a week or two. During this time focus on barefoot walking and cross-training to keep blood flow to the affected area until the pain's completely gone. Studies now suggest a lack of exercise after rest may inhibit healing.

In cases of long-term Achilles tendonitis, several new studies suggest muscle training is necessary to rehabilitate the Achilles. Also, work on rolling out your calves and Achilles with a foam roll and consider hiring a knowledgeable massage therapist to work out the knots and get things loose. Acupuncture can also help. However, only after things have loosened up should you ease back in starting with a minute or two of jogging to begin.

A last note of warning: if you ever feel a snake bite on the base of your Achilles or calf, STOP and head home slowly. You're being warned of an imminent tear ahead. Ice (10–20 minutes on and off for an hour or two), rest, then don't begin again until it feels better—typically 1 to 2 weeks.

Patellar tendonitis or pain just beneath the knees

Causes: A common problem in a shoe, though less so when barefoot. When you're running in a shoe, you likely drive force straight up through the knee, which can lead to tendonitis in the patellar tendon, the tendon connecting the lower leg to the knee. When barefoot, the condition's often caused by introducing new terrain, challenges, speed, or duration too quickly, and in particular steep uphills and any downhills. (It can also be caused by introducing weight training or balance work too quickly.)

In these cases you're asking your quadriceps to do too much work, too quickly. When your quadriceps fatigue, the load is taken up by the patellar tendon—never meant to handle the weight. (Watch how quickly you build up trail work for all knee conditions, starting with short distances once or twice a week. Trails build lateral stability and balance, but also strain weak muscles and can pull on the knees in many different ways.)

Solution: The key is rest, stretching, changing your form, and being kinder to your body. Work on rolling out the quadriceps with a foam roll to get down the tension (also massages of the quad and hamstring will help) and rest. Once the pain's gone away, build back more slowly, introduce new terrain and challenges with greater care, and run with shorter strides. If you're wearing heavy shoes, get rid of them. Heavy shoes accentuate the problem. Also, back off the gym exercises, including your one-legged balance exercises and lunges until you've built back slowly.

Chondromalacia or "runner's knee"

Causes: Felt as pain inside or beneath the knee. A grinding knee is a common problem in a shoe, where force is driven up through the knee, but very uncommon when barefoot (or out of that high-heeled, heavily cushioned shoe). However, if it's not truly bone-on-bone pain, but pulling that's causing this condition, it could be caused by imbalanced or weak hip muscles, or tight IT bands. Imbalances yank and twist your legs and knees.

Solution: Just as with patellar tendonitis, back way off, get out of your clunky footwear, strengthen imbalances, and live on a foam roll, then build back slowly. Watch your form and be careful you're not leaning forward at the waist (with your butt sticking out behind you), that you're staying light and tall on your toes, and that your feet aren't pointing out to the sides. If your feet are pointed outward, you're likely straining your knees as they won't be able to bend up and down freely. Your knees are meant to track forward, not to the sides.

Remember, weak hips or tight hip muscles can cause pain under the kneecap or your knee to track abnormally. Work on hip strength, flexibility, and muscle tension reduction by using a foam roll and tennis ball (and consider a skilled massage therapist).

IT band syndrome

Causes: A high-heeled running shoe, poor alignment, asymmetrical weaknesses, tight muscles and weak stabilizing muscles are the leading culprits. Tight and irritated illiotibial bands (the connective tissue that extends from the outside of the pelvis, over the hip and knee, and inserts just below the knee) are one of the most common, yet debilitating syndromes or injuries in running, primarily with shoes on; however, tight IT bands can still occur when barefoot. They're insidious buggers too, often coming when you feel at your best. Why? Muscle imbalances, which often grow worse as you get stronger.

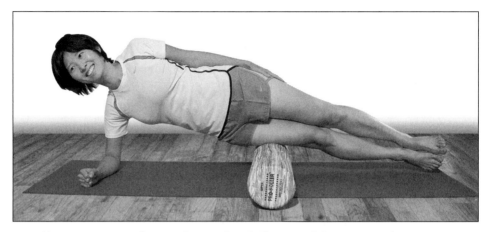

Rolling out your muscles on a foam roll or ball is one of the greatest gifts you can give yourself in the world.

Solution: The solution here is to strip off the shoes, become aware, work on alignment, and on symmetry in muscle strength, along with significant changes in stride and form (work on hip strengthening exercises and consider seeing a Franklin Method trainer or other muscle alignment specialist). Additionally, start into rocky terrain slowly whether in a shoe or out. Weak stabilizing muscles force the IT band to work overtime, as do over supportive shoes, which roll your feet to the outside. Be wary of support as you go barefoot, and build into uneven terrain slowly.

Spend substantial time rolling out your IT band on a foam roll and sitting on a tennis ball or Yamuna or RunBare ball to loosen up the muscles that attach to your hips and pelvis. Until things are better, stretch one for one—one minute on a foam roll, for example, for each minute you run, and even longer on a day off to increase blood flow and loosen things up.

Pain on the top of the knee

Causes: Tight quads or muscle imbalances. As a cyclist, speed skater, and hilly-trail–runner, I used to have overdeveloped quads relative to my hamstrings. The solution was to balance muscle strength by focusing on hamstring strength. Barefoot running also helps rebalance a body imbalanced in shoes.

Solution: Work on rolling out your hamstrings and calves, seeing a massage therapist, and working to have more balanced strength. Hit the gym to strengthen hamstrings, then learn to stride light. With a few months of easy barefoot jogging, you'll help reset your muscles and bring things back into proper balance.

Tight hamstrings and hamstring pulls

Causes: Tight hamstrings typically come from time spent in a high-heeled running shoe. They force you to run in a constant stretch. This can also occur when you carry forth your bad habits of running with your pelvis tilted forward when running bare-foot.

Solution: Work on getting your pelvis level and, of course, get out of those high-heeled shoes. Above all else, don't run hard until your hamstrings are loosened up. (Of course, never, ever, stretch tight hamstrings when they're cold before a run. It's a perfect way to help them tighten up more and get them to pull or tear on your run.)

Hip issues

Causes: Many problems are associated with the hips, from tight hips, inflammation, grinding, popping and more. Imbalanced hip strength and tight hips often get you in big trouble. The most common challenges are associated with tight hip flexors, glutes, quads, or hamstrings. Hip challenges can also certainly come from leg length discrepancies. Additionally, studies show that the hips receive almost 60 percent more torque when running in a shoe, than without.

Solution: Do away with high-heeled running shoes. They're terrible for the hips. Work to reduce tension on your hips and butts by stretching out all muscles in the area, in particular your hip flexors and glutes by using a foam roll, 5-inch inflatable Yamuna or RunBare ball, or a tennis ball. Build hip strength symmetrically with balance work and single leg exercises.

Work on proper form and make sure you're not wearing an over-supportive shoe that's rolling your feet or legs to the outside. Also watch how quickly you're building

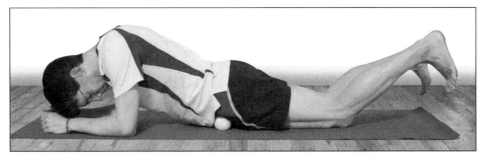

You'll find a tight rope of muscle between your groin and inner thigh. Resting on a ball here will greatly help this loosen up, helping relieve tension on your back and increasing fluidity and efficiency (not to mention speed) in your stride. Yes, you may be singing soprano as you begin to stretch here (owwww!), but it's worth it!

into trails and uneven terrain. This puts incredible stress and strain on your IT bands causing pain on the outsides of your knees and on your hips. Build up more slowly, working on uneven terrain only once or twice a week.

Also watch how you sit at work, which can significantly tighten your hips. So sit tall with your legs firmly planted on the floor and your core engaged. Consider sitting on an inflatable ball or on a balance disk on your chair.

Hips require maintenance, stretching, foam roll, and massage. The good news is that the happier your hips, the happier every part of your legs, and even your feet feel. Happy hips equal happy legs!

Groin pulls

Causes: Another common condition in shoes, particularly when over striding or when your stability is weak, but can occur when barefoot if you increase your speed too quickly or are sprinting on uneven terrain.

Solution: Build into speed, sprints, and the fast rocky stuff slowly, with no more than two days of speed a week. Groin strains can be aided with a foam roll, but are a sign you need to back off.

Side stitches

Causes: In the first mile of my first high school cross-country race I led the field. By the third I was crawling on the ground, writhing in pain. It wasn't that I went too hard, it was that my core was too weak. Stitches aren't caused by what you ate or didn't eat or drank or didn't drink. They're caused by a weak core.

Stitches are particularly common when you try to race barefoot if you haven't focused on your core as it is forced to work overtime to anchor your fast-moving legs and to support your diaphragm and lungs for proper breathing. They're also quite common if you're running on a more challenging surface than you're used to (such as chip and seal or gravel). Your core is required to do much more of the work to keep you balanced and hold proper form.

Solution: The answer to stitches is quite simple. Focus on core strength, both through Pilates-type exercises and core strengthening/balance work on a teeter board or balance device and the drills covered in earlier chapters. My favorite is one-legged work on an inflatable disk. No amount of traditional sit-ups or stomach crunches does the trick. These exercises only help you to cheat and throw your back and legs into the action. You need exercises that help you feel and isolate your core.

Additionally, holding proper form at lower speeds and very gradually working up to the fast stuff will help you keep your core engaged, keep you strong, and those stitches at bay. Work on engaging your core throughout the day, whether in the kitchen, driving, at work, sitting down, or walking around.

Stomach aches when you run

Causes: Overeating or trying new foods before or during a run (or in severe cases dehydration or overheating)

Solution: Look at what you ate and drank—and when—before you run. If you build into things slowly, you can run on much more food than you think. But you have to introduce this slowly, or you'll feel sick to your stomach. Personally, I stay away from any new foods, or foods I'm not used to exercising on, before a hard run, and always stay away from the sweet stuff or food products with chemical names I can't pronounce or understand on the food label if I'm going to be running within two and a half hours.

Sore arms

Causes: Fatigue or overuse, typically when getting into proper form or carrying heavy water bottles

Solution: This is quite common when you get into carrying your hand weights, therefore choose a minimalist shoe so you're not carrying a 14-ounce motion control boot in each hand. It's yet another reason to begin barefoot running every other day. If not, you may get tendonitis of the wrist, elbow, or even shoulder.

Sore back

Causes: A common problem when you begin running with minimalist footwear, particularly of the flexible soled varieties. It comes from not changing your form and landing too much midfoot and not high enough on your toes. Force is transmitted through your feet, knees (ouch), hips, and ultimately into your back. It can also occur if your core is very weak and forced to keep you erect. Can occur from over striding in a shoe and transmitting shock and force through the body.

Solution: First, make sure you're doing core strengthening exercises, balance exercises, or Pilates to ensure you maintain proper running form. Get tall when you run, engage that core, take shorter steps, and stay higher on your toes. This likely means backing off on the distance until you can ensure you're only running with proper form. A sore back often comes from sore calves or Achilles too. When your lower legs are sore, you often change your stride to compensate. While that seems sound, what you are actually doing is taking your Achilles and calves out of the equation as shock absorbers. This changes your form and inadvertently transmits force up through your body and into your back, shoulders, and neck. Back way off, build up the calves and Achilles, and work on that proper forefoot form. Finally, work on stretching your hips and IT bands. Tightness here pulls directly on your lower back.

Neck problems

Causes: Tends to be caused by cocking your head to one side, holding tension in your upper back and/or shoulders, wearing heavy shoes, or running with improper form, or a weak core and neck. (Also, are you running with shrugged shoulders?)

Solution: As with back challenges, work on proper form and symmetry and core strength (use this as an opportunity to try Pilates). Additionally, make sure you're running relaxed (focus on running light and easy), and that you're not carrying tension. If you can't get rid of the tension, consider a massage therapist, acupuncturist, chiropractor, or even Feldenkrais specialist to help you release the tension that's built up in your body and become stuck in your back and neck.

Breathing issues or shortness of breath

Causes: Can be caused by a weak core, bending forward too much, rolling in your shoulders (narrowing your chest, rather than bringing it up and wide), tightening up rather than relaxing, and building up speed too quickly. Of course, it can also occur from running in heavy shoes or trying to push things too much. It can also be caused by holding fear or tension in your lungs, or being afraid to take deep breaths—common in our fast-paced society. (It can also be due to asthma or conditions you want to check out with a doc. When it comes to the heart and lungs, when in doubt, check it out.)

Solution: What to do? First, if you've been diagnosed with asthma, you may benefit from practicing reverse-diaphragmatic breathing. With each breath, focus on the exhalation by pushing or squeezing in your diaphragm and blowing air out, then letting your lungs refill on their own. As a former asthmatic, I found this to be a powerful technique I learned from a book called *BreathPlay* by Ian Jackson. Cases of asthma aside, a small lung or one lung is not a limiting factor, but it's a belief that it is. If you believe you can make your lungs stronger, and find more ways to work with the air you have (gaining efficiency), then you can overcome this challenge and more.

According to Timothy Noakes, author of *The Lore of Running*, it's not how much oxygen you bring into your body that determines your ability to run, but how economical you are with the oxygen you bring in. This is good news because it means that no matter how big or how small your lungs, there's incredible room for improvement.

In addition to your traditional MD, consider alternative medicine and supplements to help relax, strengthen, and open airways. My personal favorites are garlic, onions, and other strong-smelling foods. Build up slowly, particularly into cold weather (I've fried my lungs racing in the cold), and stay aware of how you hold your chest and shoulders.

Tight jaw or sore teeth

Causes: Strangely enough, this is a common occurrence with runners. While we try to keep our mouths open for breathing, we often find ourselves clenching our jaws.

Solution: Work on running light, picturing yourself lighter than a feather, or as if you're a hot air balloon, floating into the sky with each step. The lighter and more relaxed you feel, the more your face muscles and jaws will loosen up. This visualization will not only help your running, but keep you from getting scowls or other strange lines forming on your face.

Best advice on this, focus on a smile when you run. When you're smiling, you're naturally breathing better, you're sending more endorphins to the brain (even if you're smiling when you're unhappy, your brain doesn't know it, and still releases happy drugs). Try smiling sometime when you're unhappy or if you're sore out on a run. Hold a smile for a full minute and see if you can still be as unhappy.

Foot fatigue

Causes: Even when you gradually overwork your feet, there'll be times when they feel sore.

Solution: Rest is best. If your feet are sore, particularly if there's an acute sore spot, ice your feet for 10 to 20 minutes after a workout, then elevate your feet (prop them up against a wall) to quickly reduce the inflammation. If they're still in acute pain, ice on and off for 20 minutes at a time. If there's still pain, consider a visit to a doctor. Once acute pain's gone, work to loosen things up with stretches (using a tennis ball, golf ball, or other foot stretching device).

Overall, the secret to staying healthy and running barefoot for a lifetime is to be aware, listen, build slowly, trust your intuition, work on balance, symmetry, flexibility and core strength, and focus on your form. I repeat—focus on your form. That's where everything (from speed to endurance) comes from, and if you're running symmetrically with near-perfect form, you'll not only learn to fly but you just might stay injury-free.

13

Run with Wings on Your Feet

I found [shoes] uncomfortable and after that I decided to continue running barefoot because I found it more comfortable. I felt more in touch with what was happening—I could actually feel the track.

—Zola Budd

When you're dancing from rock to rock, or footfall to footfall, watching the world go by in a blur—that's barefoot running at its best.

Whether you're just getting into the sport, are trying to heal and get going again, or want to set a new personal record, barefoot running may help you achieve your goal. And I'm here to support you 100 percent of the way.

Running barefoot is running the way nature intended, light and fast. Whether you use barefoot running as a tool to get faster in shoes, or as a means unto itself, there's no doubt in my mind, if you train barefoot, you're going to become the fastest runner you've ever been, and surprise the heck out of yourself and those around you. You'll set your own personal bests with style and grace.

When are you ready to go fast? Going fast barefoot is not something you do overnight. It's something you want to build into slowly, after building great habits, and strong feet. The faster you go, the exponentially greater the force on the feet.

Even after a 3-month transition, your feet are just getting into the game. Jogging lightly is far different than going full speed. To do this well, you need to prepare your feet. I recommend a minimum of 3 to 6 months of basic training and foot strengthening before you even think of going fast. And if you're thinking of competition, take another 3 months before you are ready to race.

Go Slow to Go Fast

Remember our mantra about going slow to go fast. You may not race this season. However, if you need to race fast, for now, do it in a minimalist shoe. As for barefoot racing, going slow now is investing in a faster future.

As runners, we're impatient, and we want it all, and want it yesterday. The good news is, you can have it all. You can PR time after time after time. But those personal records are going to have to wait until tomorrow. First you must build your foundation, then you can build your house. Go slow and be the tortoise. Next year will be your best season ever.

Let's look at getting into speed, and then into racing.

Speed is much more demanding on your body for these reasons:

- **The Landing Force Is Far Greater.** You need a much stronger and more flexible foot to handle speed. When your foot's strong, it'll be the greatest coil-spring in the world. But until then, it can turn to mush at speed, slamming down with an instant overuse injury, or worse—a fracture.

- **Different Forces Are Involved.** As you increase speed, your stride starts to change. You may bring the outside of your foot down first, and you'll get far more stress on the sides of your feet as you handle turns and undulations at speed. This means growing the feet stronger to handle forces they never encountered when going slow.

- **Your Skin Faces New Challenges.** When you're going fast, you're landing differently and using your toes differently. Additionally, surfaces that once appeared smooth and soft when slow become coarse and challenging. Perhaps your feet will slide more, scuffing things up fast, or new parts of your foot will make contact with the ground, chewing them up as well (the tips of your toes and inside of your big toe). In general, skin that's ready for slow jogging must strengthen anew for speed.

- **More Demands on Core Muscles.** You need a stronger core to keep proper form when the going gets fast. In fact, if you haven't put much effort into strengthening your core, on race day, you may find yourself doubled over with intense stitches in your side.

When you get into speed, the most important thing you can do is listen to your body. Ask yourself the following questions:

- *Is my body ready for a speed workout?* I once did a speed workout after I'd been sick for a few weeks. I'd been working late nights on the book and not getting enough rest. It was the first time I'd been sick in years, but I didn't want to lose my strength and speed. Unfortunately, I wasn't thinking clearly and didn't practice what I preach.

I ignored the warning signs and did a fast workout (on a treadmill, no less!) and in 8 minutes I'd torn my feet up, taking nearly 3 full months to recover. In a desire to stay fast, I didn't listen to my body. Because I was weak, I couldn't maintain my form and landed funny, quickly tearing my feet apart. The moral of the story is if you can't maintain form, don't even begin.

- *Am I maintaining proper form or is my body fatiguing?* If you find your form changing or falling apart, don't be afraid to stop or head for home (even if you're in a race). You need to be incredibly aware of your body and need to feel your form. This requires incredible vigilance.

Michael's 8 Rules for Building into Speed

When you feel you are ready, follow these rules to help you transform from a strong, steady-state runner to a barefoot jackrabbit.

1. **Think Quality Over Quantity.** Begin with 1 to 2 fast runs per week. Never do more than 3. Less is more for speed work. Much better to have 2 great workouts a week with plenty of recovery, than 3 where you're tearing yourself up. Speed comes from training fresh legs.

2. **Run Up Hills.** For your first month of speed work, run hills rather than flats. This minimizes impact to your body, while helping build form, feet, and in particular strong skin for speed. Run the uphills fast, then travel slowly downhill and home (downhills are the hardest, ease into downhills infinitesimally slowly, see the chapter on exploring terrain for more on downhills).

3. **Let Your Stride Be Your Guide.** Never exceed the speed of your feet or the speed of your form. Your form should remain rock solid and your stride intact, no matter what the speed. If your stride changes, for instance, if you typically land nice and high on the forefoot—but at speed you rush and slap down flat—you're going too fast. Instead, back down to a speed where you can land the same way, then work on building up (over many workouts) your speed from there. Here's an example: if your stride's great at 7-minute miles, but the minute you do 6:30 your heels are smacking the ground, back off to where you can maintain your stride such as 6:50 for a workout or two. Then go 6:45, 6:40, and so on until you're way below 6:30, but with perfect form that won't bite you. Form trumps speed *every time*. Build perfect form and it'll keep you

safe, no matter what the speed. But force the pace and watch your form break down, and your body will soon follow.

4. **Lay Off the Goals.** Goals may be motivators, but they can get you into a world of trouble. It's best to let go of the outcome and let the speed come naturally. For instance, don't say you need a 7-minute pace in 2 weeks or a fast 10K next month. Done this way, you're more able and likely to listen to your body—and never to push it too far. This doesn't mean you can't or won't go fast, or will never win the race or PR. It just means your speed will come more naturally, and with a better foundation, keeping you fit, healthy, and fast as you progress.

5. **Think Speed or Duration.** They're inversely proportional. Raise one, lower the other. For instance, if you pick up the pace, you must back off the distance. If not, you're liable to overdo things.

6. **Recover.** Give yourself plenty of recovery. As you get into speed, cut back on the miles and give yourself plenty of recovery. Never do speed work 2 days in a row, and never before fully rested. Instead, rest well, go light in between speed days, and let your body fully recover.

7. **Careful on the Treadmill.** Don't get sucked into the need for speed. Remember, treadmills change the force dynamics of your stride. You must decelerate your foot with each step (or brake) in order to catch the belt. This force can bite you badly, if you're not ready. Also, due to your close proximity to the control panel and cushioning of a treadmill, your stride inherently changes. So build in slowly (start with a few minutes at speed and no more, then build up a minute per workout), watch yourself in a mirror to check your form, and realize the dangers involved.

8. **Careful on the Track.** Tracks are ideal for speedwork—and for overuse injuries. Make sure you let go of the goal and use the track sparingly to begin. Like a treadmill, a cushioned track can be especially unforgiving. Alternate directions, maintain proper form, and build in incredibly slowly (a lap or two at speed and no more to begin, then increase one lap per workout, every other day or less to begin).

Running Your Best Race

If you'd like to try out your new stride and new feet, you'll amaze yourself with your speed. If you're interested in racing, then this section's for you. Here's specific information to help you race barefoot or in your new minimalist shoes.

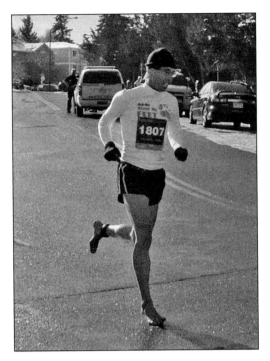

What do 24 degrees, rock salt, snow, and ice have in common? The 2009 Colder Boulder 5K in Boulder, Colorado. Racing's fun, but make sure you keep it safe. Michael passes runners and can't wait to get inside to get warm.

Shoes? Yes or no?

Do you want to race in shoes? It's a big decision. Training barefoot makes you stronger and faster, whether or not you're in shoes. Kenyans and Ethiopians, some of the best barefoot runners in the world, almost always race in shoes—at least in the West, either due to sponsors or conditions. And Haile Gebrselassie, who grew up running barefoot, uses his barefoot stride while wearing shoes to dominate the world at most long distances.

Racing in shoes doesn't make you weak and often protects the feet. Personally, however, I like the additional challenge and learning that comes from feeling the ground as I race. But there's no right or wrong decision. We're all just out there to have fun and go fast. And if you're looking for a PR, unless you've developed feet of steel, chances are it'll come while running in a shoe.

Remember, too, even if you've been training barefoot, it's a whole different game to enter a race barefoot. Everything becomes more difficult, at least initially.

Think specificity. If you choose to race in shoes, you need to train for speed in shoes too. You'll need to do half of your speed work in shoes. Always do the first half of your runs barefoot, then the second part in shoes. If you do the reverse, your feet may be soft and sweaty from shoes, then get torn up on the ground. Additionally, make sure you train in the shoes you'll race in, and if the race is a half-marathon or longer, do at least one long shod run per week. If not, your feet won't be ready.

The longer you've gone barefoot, the more I'd recommend the most minimal shoe you can find. However, while I love training in moccasins or socklike shoes such as the Sockwa or Feelmax, for race day, I'd recommend a racing flat. Consider the Asics Piranha, Mizuno Wave Universe, or your favorite racing flat. They have less flexibility than a sock-type shoe, but more protection; and for racing, they're incredibly fast.

But for me, I love racing without shoes. If you do too, you'll find fun and excitement to see the look on people's faces as you dance on by without shoes. You feel lighter, freer, and as long as you're not on a sharp surfaced road, you'll feel better too.

●°°°₀ FOOT NOTE

Tri and Stay Dry

If you're a triathlete, make sure you keep your feet dry on race day. Consider filling your cycling shoes with a centimeter of climber's chalk in advance to dry your feet for the run. Also look into exceptionally well-ventilated cycling shoes (triathlon shoes tend to be better than cycling ones, and are wider too). Then, if you're going to run in footwear, make sure they breathe well. If they don't, you'll be tearing up the strong skin you've worked so hard to get.

Steps to Race Day

Racing barefoot is a grand experiment. Go in without expectations, just to have fun and play and to learn.

In planning to race, follow this advice:

- **Don't Plan on Fast Times for Now.** If you love a particular race or course, and it'll break your heart to go slower, factor that into the equation.

- **Start with Short Distance Races.** Even if you're a marathoner, pick a shorter distance to start. Ideally, start with 5Ks and work yourself back up. Both your skin and feet may not be ready for the challenge of a long race barefoot. Better to get a bit of speed first, then build in the endurance later. This'll also prevent you from tearing things up and being stuck out on a course barefoot.

  There's an expression I learned from track racing: Easier to go slow than to go fast. This means it's easier to build endurance after you've built speed. When you start with speed first, you gain proper form and strength in your feet and muscles, then carry that form with you to the longer events.

  Most professional runners follow this format. For example, when world-record-holding runner Haile Gebrselassie got started, he raced 5Ks and shorter, gradually working his way up to marathons. Usain Bolt, Jamaican sprinter and 3-time Olympic gold medalist, is starting with the 100- and 200-meter dashes, but according to his coach, Glen Mills, will eventually progress to the 400-meter race. Work on speed and form now, then distance later on, just like the fast guys.

- **Pre-Run the Course.** Some courses are just not barefoot friendly. If the course is running through cactus and sage, or heavy chip and sealed roads, you may wish to forgo the race. Always check the course in advance to know what you're getting into.

From Starting Gun to Finish Line: A Checklist

Pre-race day

- **Timing Chip.** If you need to wear a timing chip, check it out in advance, or better yet, ask the organizers in advance. They may need you to wear a special chip they can provide, or need you to do a special set-up. In general, most chips will do quite well when strapped to the leg just above the ankle, even if the organizer is not sure it will. However, be forewarned that it may not work. In one race I had to dash back and across the line with chip in hand.

- **Throw Out the Watch.** Can you run your first few races without a watch? If so, you're far more likely to let go of the outcome and let your feet do their dance.

Race day

- **Stay Well Hydrated Before You Race.** Hydration helps keep your muscles loose and your joints moving smoothly. Pre-race hydration, particularly days leading up to the race (and the critical night before) are important to feel at your best. Since your feet must do all the work, the better hydrated you are, the better you'll feel.

- **When in Doubt, Bring Your Hand Weights.** If you're out on the course and your skin gives way, you can get yourself into a lot of trouble, fast. Consider bringing protection along, just in case. Even something as minimal as Sockwas can help if you get yourself in trouble. And if you're racing on the trails, bring shoes just to be safe, or for steep or rocky downhills. These can be lifesavers when the going gets tough.

- **Keep Yourself Warm before the Race.** Bring warm-up shoes and warm clothes. If your legs and feet are cold before you race, you'll struggle early on. So keep yourself warm and walk around in shoes or at least sandals, until it's time to warm up.

Start slow and warm up your feet and legs well. Since your feet are your shoes, you need them at their best, from stride one. I recommend wearing free-moving shoes such as Feelmax footwear as you begin to warm up (they'll help your feet get warm and loose faster), then strip them off.

The race

- **Start Near the Front or Off to the Side.** While it's unlikely to be an issue, every now and again someone gets stepped on. By starting out of the way, you're less likely to get stomped. Now out on the course, that's another story. Always run aware.

- **Look for the Path.** When you begin racing you'll find your feet do better on some surfaces than others. Look for these surfaces on the course. For instance, if there's a smooth painted centerline, be there. Or if a clean gutter's smoother than the road, run there as well. If the sidewalk's smooth and legal to run on, consider it, even if it's 10 feet away. You may find the smoother surface helps you run much faster than the rougher road you're trodding on.

- **Maintain Form.** If your stride starts to fall apart, back off. Best to go slower and focus on being light. There's no need to hurt yourself to go fast; instead, consider this preparation for faster races to come.

- **Keep Your Strides Short.** Don't try matching strides with shod runners. Instead keep yourself tall and with your roadrunner-like feet whirring around at 180-plus short strides per minute.

- **Keep Your Arms Up.** Don't drop your arms, no matter what. This is something to work on in all your speed workouts too. If you drop your arms, you're dropping your legs, and twisting your upper body, making yourself more injury prone, and far less efficient. Work on keeping your spring-loaded chicken wings up high into the sky, with your chest pressed slightly forward letting gravity do the work.

- **Be the Observer and Experiment.** Consider each race a class at school, using each to tinker and improve. Step back from the race and watch yourself and others. Observe your form, breathing, technique, stride, mental attitude, and even what you're thinking about during the race. The more you learn about yourself, the better you'll be.

- **Stay in a Place of Gratitude.** It's easy for our egos to get the best of us on race day. However, we run safe and fast when we're present, not when we're focused on ego. To keep the ego at bay, stay in a place of gratitude. When you're thankful for the run, or the race, or for your health, or even for the runners around you, you'll stay present. This keeps you safe and happy and helps you turn your best times. (I like to give thanks, just before the race and throughout. If you're aware enough, you can use your entire race as a running meditation.)

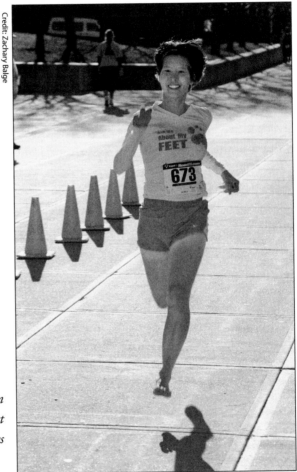

Credit: Zachary Balge

As a former 400 runner early in high school, Jessica's favorite part of the race was, is, and always will be the sprint finish.

Post-race

- **Cool Down Fast.** Get off your feet as quickly as possible. If it's cold, get inside and throw on warm clothes fast, and if it's hot, hydrate. Above all else, don't hang out race-side without recovering. Ideally, if your feet are toast, ice them and your calves for 10 to 20 minutes after a race, while propping your legs up to let fluids drain. Mingling après-race is great, but don't neglect your recovery.

Racing Dietary Dos and Don'ts

To keep yourself healthy and well fueled, make sure you eat a good meal several hours before your race. Don't worry about carbo loading or stuffing yourself with carbs for days before a race. Doing so tends to make your stomach sick, and changing your diet unnaturally stresses your body, eliminating any possible gain.

Don't down sugary drinks within 20 to 30 minutes of a race, as they'll crash your blood sugar, just when you need it most. And if you're eating sugary stuff during a race (such as gel packs), try to eat those with the most complex carbohydrates you can, and take one pack every 20 minutes after you start to keep yourself from bonking or your blood sugar spiking, then crashing through the floor.

Never experiment with a new race diet (or equipment) on race day.

It's especially important to refuel and rehydrate immediately after a race in order to adequately replenish your fuel stores, particularly muscle glycogen. Refuel quickly with high-quality protein, carbs, and fat, beginning within the first 45 minutes after your race or hard run. Eating early and rehydrating well helps refuel muscles and repair damage.

Racing barefoot is fast and fun. We're light, free, and boy can we go! As with everything else, the trick is to build in slowly and be smart. Listen to your body. It will never steer you wrong. Once you've given it time and you're ready to go, explore, test things out, and try out your new wings.

Perhaps you'll PR, or fly across your local trail. Maybe you'll dance through ultras or smoke a local 5K. Who knows, maybe, just maybe, you'll be the one who'll medal at the Olympics. The sky's the limit when it comes to barefoot running, but stay humble, follow the wings on your feet, and watch yourself soar.

PART IV

Discovering and Rediscovering the Joy of Barefoot Running at Any Age

Show me a man with both feet on the ground and I'll show you a man who can't get his pants on.

—Joe E. Lewis

14

Barefoot Children

This little piggy went to market.
This little piggy stayed at home.
This little piggy has roast beef,
This little piggy had none.
And this little piggy cried
"Wee! Wee! Wee! I'm barefoot!"
All the way home.

—Mother Goose as interpreted by Jessica Lee

How many times do parents tell their kids, "Put on your shoes!" Or that they'll get hurt running around barefoot? What if we rethink all that?

A lifetime of healthy running begins with running barefoot as a child. Children naturally love the feeling of going barefoot, running through the grass, playing on a beach, or running in soft dirt. Kenyans, Ethiopians, and so many other third-world countries have such incredible runners and with infinitely fewer foot and running injuries—all because they started the kids barefoot and kept them barefoot as long as possible. Running barefoot may be what gives children those springs on their feet and stronger legs.

I've known many runners, such as Hendrick Maako, one of the fastest marathoners out there, who grew up running barefoot in South Africa. As Hendrick put it, "My feet were so strong back then, but it all changed once I got my first sponsor and was given shoes. I got soft."

It's a shame, perhaps almost a crime, that we force kids today to stay in shoes. We stunt the development of their feet and make them feel it's unsafe. Study after study suggests how much stronger children's feet get, how much the bones and musculature develop from walking and running barefoot, and how much the nerve endings develop in kids by going barefoot too.

Barefoot running or walking, particularly in children, not only strengthens the feet, but prevents maladaptation (deformity) due to shoes. It helps their toes, arches, ankles, Achilles, shins, knees, hips, the back (core), and more grow incredibly strong. A child who runs barefoot is building a strong, healthy body for a lifetime. He or she gains greater balance, greater bone density, joint strength, neural pathways, and even greater blood flow and circulation. Barefoot running also helps build a body that will be injury, fatigue, and disease resistant for years to come.

Whether your child's 4 or 14, he or she can still become a fantastic barefoot runner. Why would you want that? For a lifetime of health. Running, playing, and exploring barefoot helps a child learn, grow, and be a natural kid again. A child who enjoys running becomes an adult who will likely always take care of his or her body and grow up calmer, more independent, and more in tune with nature.

Even if your child has been in shoes all the way into teen years, it's not too late to make substantial changes. Though their feet may be full grown, they're still in the developmental years. Teenagers' feet likely haven't weakened and fully deformed the way adults' feet have. Moreover, they still have growth hormones coursing through their veins to help them change and build incredibly strong, healthy feet, legs, bones, and joints.

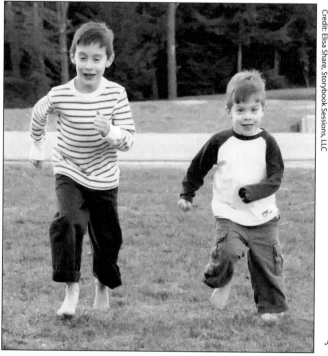

Credit: Elisa Share, Storybook Sessions, LLC

Children were born to run and play barefoot. They have a natural fore-foot stride.

Let's learn how to help our kids develop their full physical potential, all by taking off their shoes or keeping them out of shoes to begin with.

No Running on the Playground

I remember giving a talk on attention deficit disorder in Howard County, Maryland, at a local school. To my dismay, I saw these signs at a school:

"NO RUNNING ON THE PLAYGROUND"

No wonder our kids are so challenged today. We're completely unplugging them from both nature and who they are. Our children were meant to run and play. However, in an effort to protect our children and keep them from harm, we've kept them from their true nature. Just as we strap shoes on our children to keep them from stepping on sharp objects, or stubbing a toe, we've kept them from running and playing the way we did as kids. Some schools have cut recess entirely or done away with PE classes.

But in an effort to protect them, we're likely doing far more harm than good. So concludes Richard Louv, author of *Last Child in the Woods*, who says that by taking our kids out of nature, they're suffering from what he terms *nature deficit disorder* or attention deficit disorder–like symptoms. He believes this is caused by being stuck indoors, in front of a PlayStation, or a TV, and not having the time to play outdoors the way kids once did.

Nature deficit disorder is the term used to describe a lack of attention and focus, memory, impulsivity control, and anger management issues, some of the very traits kids get by being outside, independent, and playing in nature. I believe these traits are further exacerbated by being insulated from and not feeling the ground.

Barefoot Benefits for Children

- **Strong Toes Equal Strong Tots.** It all begins with the foot. If we have healthy feet, the rest of the body will follow. Fortunately, strengthening the feet is easy, particularly for kids. The younger they start, the better. Catch them earlier enough and keep them out of a shoe, and they'll have the best, healthiest, most natural feet, legs, and bodies in the world.

  Babies' feet have strong, healthy toes that are as nimble and dexterous as our fingers. There's a beautiful spread between the first and second toe, and each toe spreads out, perfect to act as a spring and launching pad for their newly discovered walking and running attempts. Keep kids out of shoes, and these feet stay in their natural shape, strong, wide, and with a powerful arch. Put them in shoes, however, and the toes get squashed together, the arch goes flat and weak, and the foot loses its springlike character.

Studies show that if you start children barefoot (or keep them out of their shoes as much as possible), their feet get stronger, more supple, wider, and gain a more stable forefoot. Their feet stay warmer, they gain stronger connective tissues and muscles from their feet, ankles, knees, hip, and back (and they have better posture than their shod counterparts).

• **Waking Up "Eyes" to Better Feel the Earth.** Touching the ground and thus waking up the nerve endings on the bottom of their feet, children become more aware of their surroundings and become wired to sense more. In essence, it's like waking up a new sense or talent. The earlier it's discovered and utilized, the more this awareness can be strengthened and grown. Consider this process to be somewhat like waking up the "eyes" on the bottom of your children's feet—helping them be better in touch with the earth, better balanced, more stable, and able to run like the wind, and better feel the world around them.

• **Becoming King of the Hill.** By giving kids a chance to be outside, to feel the ground, and to play and connect with nature in an unstructured way, we're giving them the greatest opportunity in the world to de-stress and be kids again. That in turn has an incredibly calming and empowering effect.

Playing in the woods and feeling the ground or feeling nature gives kids a feeling of being the King of the Hill. In today's world, we often rob our children of the opportunity to feel empowered. This makes children more fearful, and takes away the self-esteem they need to overcome life's greatest hurdles. By letting a child play free, feel the ground, and become one with nature, you're giving a child the chance to spread his or her wings, to explore the world and let his or her imagination soar.

• **Habla "Coordination."** Helping a child feel the ground and using the hard wiring of the neural connections that grow is like teaching a child a foreign language. The earlier we do it, the more neural pathways there are for learning even more new languages, for memorization skills, and so much more sensory awareness. The better children are able to walk, run, or hike, the more capable and better balanced they will be at so many physical endeavors and (life) activities.

• **Smarter Than the Prey.** In many parts of the word, persistence hunters continue to chase and track animals till exhaustion (the animal, not the hunter). However, it's not uncommon for these hunters to occasionally lose the tracks of their prey. This doesn't mean it's game over for the hunters (no pun intended). These hunters will feel the ground and can "sense" where the animal has gone. This sense comes from wiring the mind to connect to the earth and nature's cues. Children can wire this connection, strength, and innate talent far more readily and profoundly than adults. When you enable children to develop these skills naturally, you help cultivate more intelligent and intuitive children.

Think of the brain as something that's very plastic, fluid, changeable, and loves to grow. Children are growing hundreds of thousands of new neurons daily. Touching the ground is stimulating such brain growth. It's akin to teaching the brain a new language or a new form of creative expression, such as music. Over a lifetime our connection to the earth can become incredibly strong or unbelievably weak.

- **Trigger Points and Reflexology.** Studies have shown that stimulation from the ground is amazingly effective at reducing tension and aiding with relaxation. Acupressure and reflexology have many health benefits, from lowering blood pressure, to reducing anxiety and depression, and to aiding the immune system—all great benefits for our children.

"Getting grounded" in this way has two positive health benefits. First, by reducing the static electric charge on our bodies, we are purging our body of harmful free radicals that create a whole host of physical ailments. By draining these electrons, it's like giving your child a massive dose of instantly absorbed antioxidant vitamins. Antioxidants help reduce inflammation, prevent disease, and boost the immune system.

By encouraging your child to go barefoot each day, you help your child recharge the mind and sync with the earth to put them back in the zone for focused, concentrated studies, anxiety free.

- **Going with the Flow to the Feet.** When your foot's not in a shoe, the muscles of the foot have to do all of the work to support your body. Because of this, the muscles of the foot need more blood flow. To give the feet the blood flow it needs, the body develops better circulation (arteries, capillaries, and veins) to nourish the muscles of the feet. Therefore a child's feet and legs get better circulation and naturally stay much warmer. As counterintuitive as it sounds, getting children out of shoes can make their feet warmer.

- **No More Cold Feet.** In a preliminary study, researchers discovered feeling the ground and its temperature may give the body more information to help regulate skin and body temperature. In a sense, when the feet can't feel the ground, the body is running blind, unsure about the temperature of the environment, and therefore how to stay warm. But when the feet touch the ground, it's like the blindfold's been removed and the body can sense the heat or the coolness all around. It helps the body (mind-body connection) learn to better regulate its temperature and to become more efficient. If the feet are always in contact with a cool ground, the body will learn to keep the skin warmer to protect the body—thus affecting the internal thermostat, the efficiency of the heat regulation system, and even the body's metabolism itself.

●°°₀ FOOT NOTE

Barefoot in the Cold

In his book *Indian Running*, Peter Nabokov talks about the Navajo tradition of having kids roll in the first or second snow of the year in order to build resistance to the cold and strengthen their immune systems. It turns out, there's good reason for this. Although you don't want to risk your child getting frostbite, studies are showing that exposing your children's feet to the cold may help their bodies adapt to the cold and better regulate skin and internal temperatures.

In a provisional study done in Japan, researchers concluded that "young children with barefoot habituation might show more effective cold adaptation of metabolic type than those without the habituation do, by keeping their skin temperatures higher even in the cold and enhancing metabolic rate."

Barefoot in the Heat

Who can forget those quick dashes across hot pavement on a hot summer's day? Or the hot swimming pool decks in the days before flip-flops and Crocs?

Native peoples such as the Aborigines in Australia handle the most incredible desert heat barefoot, because they started walking on hot surfaces as children. Hot pavement's toasty, but only in the beginning. While hot pavement can burn children's feet if exposed too much too soon, their feet adapt faster than adult feet. If they do a little bit at a time, children's feet quickly adapt to the heat.

While they'd like to let pain be their guide, kids often don't think ahead, and if they head out barefoot without a pair of shoes, they can get in trouble quickly. Best advice: monitor their early runs in the heat. Better yet, keep them outdoors year round. In this way, when the weather increasingly heats up, they'll acclimate gradually as well.

The Danger of Footwear

A child's feet are incredibly flexible, which can get them into trouble if a parent's not careful. Because the feet are so flexible, they're easy to squeeze into ill-fitting shoes and will even take the shape of these shoes over time.

Foot expert, Dr. Michael Nirenberg explains, "The downside of such a flexible foot is that if parents choose the wrong shoes or footwear for their children, they could create a deformity for their child."

According to Dr. William Rossi, author of at least 8 books on the foot, due to footwear, "Foot defects and weakening begin at age 3 and progressively increase. Starting at age 6, it is impossible to find five straight toes on shoe-wearing children."

Tight-fitting shoes and shoes with a strong in-flare (the banana-shaped curve discussed in the chapter on minimalist shoes) force a child's big toe in, creating bunions, calluses, corns, and more by the time they are adults. It prevents the toes from working naturally and, since 18 of the 19 muscles of the foot are connected to the toes, greatly weakens the toes in the process.

In addition to being soft and flexible, a child's foot adapts incredibly well to its external environments. If a child is stuck in a shoe—or even worse a shoe with arch support—the foot doesn't have to work, so the ligaments, tendons, muscles, and bones get weak and rigid and the foot loses circulation. Instead, if the child runs and plays barefoot on uneven surfaces and terrain, these same structures will quickly strengthen and gain flexibility and better circulation.

Shoes Can Harm Your Child's Feet

Researchers are weighing in on the damage shoes can cause when worn by children. In one study, scientists compared the feet of Americans who had been wearing shoes all their lives with African natives who had never worn shoes. The big difference was in the big toe. Americans showed a surprising number of deformed big toes and bunions caused, the researchers thought, by shoes curving inward—perhaps as a concession to style and to make feet seem more slender. Those pointy toes haven't done anyone a favor. The natives' feet showed a straight big toe and no bunions.

The arch is the greatest natural shock absorber in the world. Researchers Rao and Joseph examined 2,300 Indian children between the ages of 4 and 13. Their results showed that children who grew up in shoes were more than 3 times as likely to have flat feet than those out of shoes. Their conclusion: shoes (particularly those with closed toes) negatively affected the growth of a normal arch. "We suggest that children should be encouraged to play unshod and that slippers and sandals are less harmful than closed-toe shoes," they said in their study published in the *Journal of Bone and Joint Surgery.*

Note: This also means keeping a child out of socks, particularly tight-fitting ones as much as possible. These socks will also bind the foot, force the toes together, and cause deformities of the foot as well as keep the foot sweaty and moist. In the winter, if warmth is necessary, seek soft-lined moccasins or booties.

Chinese foot binding seems so abhorrent, but how much of a different outcome are our shoes creating when you think about it in light of these studies?

Footwear for Children

You probably marvel at your baby's little plump, soft and incredibly flexible feet. A baby's feet are well-cushioned with fat until we put them in a shoe. And according Dr. Michael Nirenberg, baby's feet should be kept out of shoes for as long as possible. As a child grows and ages, "due to everyday walking—not to mention, perhaps tight fitting shoes—that fat will wear away allowing our foot bones and their rough edges to dig into our skin, often causing corns, calluses, blisters and other painful conditions."

Leading doctors and podiatrists recommend keeping children out of shoes until they're at least beginning to walk, if not longer. As Dr. Nirenberg recommends: "Don't be in a hurry to buy shoes for your child; wait until your children begin to walk, usually at 11 to 15 months of age. Even then, the most important thing to do is *keep shoes off your child's feet as much as possible.* I cannot emphasize this enough! The best 'shoes' for your children is no shoes!"

The fact of the matter is kids can't go barefoot in all activities. Whether it's climbing, dance, or soccer, they may have to be in a shoe. But you want to be careful about the kind of shoe they wear.

For sports, make sure they have as wide a shoe as possible. While tight, narrow shoes may be preferred by instructors or coaches, they will cause harmful effects on children's feet. A tight ballet slipper or dance shoe, for instance, can do permanent damage. We've seen many dancers' feet that look as if they've been through a war zone before they're even 18.

For other sports where cleats are involved, minimalist shoes aren't an option either. Again, look for something that's wide and close to the ground and flexible. However, don't leave your children unprotected. If other children will be wearing cleats, make sure the upper is stiff enough to provide protection.

When it comes to climbing, see if you can start your child without shoes. Indigenous people around the world have and still climb this way, and their feet get incredibly strong and nimble. Instead of trying to force their feet into tight shoes, they use their toes to grip and climb. Just watch the native Tagbanuas of Northern Palawan in the Philippines to see what I mean. Their toes become as strong and nimble as their fingers.

Many climbing gyms and walls allow barefoot climbing. However, if shoes are a must, don't get the narrowest ones, and get them out of shoes the minute they're off the rock. Better yet, consider a minimalist shoe, but with good sticky rubber. One of the best free-climbers in the world, Jyothi Raj, known as the Indian Spiderman or the Monkey King, wears a regular minimalist shoe when he's not climbing barefoot.

Hey, Coach, Try This

If we can train high school coaches to work with their athletes barefoot, we'll build stronger, less injury-prone runners. If we can teach our young future track stars and distance runners how to run safely and efficiently with proper form, not only will we create a whole new generation of super athletes (and finally be competitive on the world stage again at distance running) but we'll help kids, from the slowest to the fastest to enjoy running and be able to run happy and injury-free, for life.

Try these barefoot training tips: Whether you're coaching high school, junior high, or even elementary school kids, introduce them to barefoot running slowly. Start kids on AstroTurf or grass and focus on form. Do not start them with barefoot sprints. Have them begin with a 100-yard jog down an infield, then come back scrunching their toes. Just do that a few times and build up from there. After building for a month or two, have them run barefoot on a track, light and easy. Additionally, work on getting them into minimalist footwear. Mizuno and Asics, among others, have minimalist track shoes and cross-country shoes that sell for $50 or less.

Countless parkour (street acrobatic) athletes also use minimalist or flat shoes. They tend to be heavier than running flats with more rubber on the bottom and the sides but close to the ground. Without an elevated heel or cushioning, they allow the climber or acrobat to feel the urban terrain.

Barefoot-like shoes for kids

Studies show the best footwear for children are not the cute, stiff, leather baby shoes we're most familiar with, nor perhaps the favorite fashion models preferred by your kids and their friends.

The best choices are loose-fitting, flexible shoes made with breathable materials and with thin soles very close to the ground. More like moccasins. Many companies have been jumping on the minimalist, flexible shoe movement for children. Around the longest are Preschoolians, Robeez, and SoftStar, which specialize in barefoot-like flexible footwear for children.

Flexible footwear will allow your child's foot to move naturally and to feel the ground, strengthen the feet, and maintain balance. The foot should not be restricted in any way so that it may move and function as naturally as possible.

Cushioning is not necessary or the main concern, as the forces generated by a child when he or she is small are very low.

Researchers in one recent study said, "The child's foot is clearly distinct from the adult foot in its functional anatomy and ability to cope with pressure … Small children should have a sports shoe, which is as flexible as their own foot. The small impact forces during their sports activities make extra cushioning superfluous."

At the same time, breathability is essential to prevent mold and fungus from growing, and to keep the skin dry and healthy. Above all else, make sure your child's toes have plenty of room to spread and move, with a minimum of a finger's width in the front of the shoes between the toes and the end. While children's feet grow fast, never have them wear the shoes until they're snug. Keep an eye on your child's shoe size. They can outgrow shoes much faster than they wear them out. If the child can't wiggle his or her toes, it's time for new shoes.

Make sure they do not have a strong curve by the big toe, which may force the toe in. If the shoes look banana shaped and stiff, avoid them at all costs.

For older children, you can get away with adult minimalist shoes. One great suggestion is Tai Chi or martial arts shoes. They look like your grandpa's slippers (sorry kids), though some are a bit more fashionable, and they let children's feet fully move (just look at Jackie Chan), allow them to feel the ground, and are low and flat. If this doesn't work for your child, have them go hunting for shoes with you.

In the vast majority of cases, children should not be in orthotics, particularly when they're young. Experts now believe that corrective shoes or devices may not do much correction at all. Instead the majority of foot deformities among young children work themselves out naturally over time. Perhaps it's because they have such soft and flexible feet when they're young. Additionally, studies show that wearing support weakens a child's foot and may prevent the development of a strong arch.

Some children, however, may need support or a corrective device. If a corrective device is recommended for your child, seek a second opinion from a podiatrist who believes in barefoot running. There are many out there, and the numbers are growing.

Playtime Barefoot Activities

Imagine finger painting with your toes. That's the kind of fun you can have while introducing your children to "barefoot time" every day.

When your children are young, work to build the dexterity and strength of their feet by encouraging barefoot time each day. This can go beyond barefoot running and walking time to include barefoot games, and even art and dexterity work with the feet.

Here are some examples of artwork children can try with their toes. However, anything they can do with the fingers, they can try with their toes. Well-known famous painters have no hands, and people have even flown airplanes with no hands, so literally, the sky's the limit.

Exercises

Art with Feet. A variation on finger painting. Use a paintbrush grasped in the toes like the famous armless artist Simona Atzori. Or try molding something with clay or Play-Doh (fantastically messy but a ton of fun).

Games for Feet. Play pick-up games with the feet, such as picking up marbles or jacks. For a more advanced version, use feet to pick up and build things with Legos. Another variation: Throwing games with the feet, such as Frisbees or even sticks like the kick-stick racing once popular with Native American children.

Exploratory Exercises. Blindfolded, have children touch different objects with their feet to try and identify them. For a fun-tastic outdoor activity, have children go into a backyard or playground blindfolded (do this in a safe location with supervision) and have them describe the surfaces they're touching with their feet.

Activities That Strengthen the Feet. Sign your children up for gymnastics, modern dance, children's yoga, and circus arts. They'll exercise their brains and their feet.

Follow the Leader (Dexterity Exercises). Play Follow the Leader barefoot where you must step exactly where the leader has stepped (over grass, safe obstacles, and other tactile surfaces). A good friend, Paul Weppler, submitted this game: Kids throw down 6-inch diameter pieces of carpet over an obstacle course. They then try jumping barefoot from one piece of carpet to the next without touching the ground.

If your baby is still barefoot, work to keep him or her that way. And if they're back in shoes, set up a time and place to go barefoot. Either way, there are times they'll need shoes, so make sure they're always in flexible footwear that allows natural movement and room for unencumbered growth.

There's nothing more natural than a child running barefoot, dancing through the grass. It doesn't just strengthen their feet, but sets them up for a lifetime of great health. It keeps their senses awake, helps build stronger bones, muscles, ligaments, and tendons, gives them greater balance, and kindles a special bond with nature.

15

Barefoot Seniors Turn Back the Clock

There is a road in the hearts of all of us, hidden and seldom traveled,
which leads to an unknown, secret place.
The old people came literally to love the soil,
and they sat or reclined on the ground with a feeling of
being close to a mothering power.
Their teepees were built upon the earth
and their altars were made of earth.
The soul was soothing, strengthening, cleansing and healing.
That is why the old Indian still sits upon the earth instead of
propping himself up and away from its life-giving forces.
For him, to sit or lie upon the ground is to be able to think more deeply
and to feel more keenly. He can see more clearly into the mysteries of
life and come closer in kinship to other lives about him.

—Chief Luther Standing Bear

Want the secret to eternal health? Take your shoes off. Whether you're an avid runner, average walker, or struggling to stay on your feet, taking off your shoes can help.

Any time spent barefoot helps regenerate nerves, stimulate bone growth, increase circulation, and lay down new bone. Add the benefits of strengthening your heart and lungs, while decreasing blood pressure, and you've found the fountain of youth in your feet.

Seniors can reap incredible benefits with barefoot living. But age also presents its own set of challenges. That's why it's essential for this demographic to start slowly. But no matter the age, no matter how soft your feet, you can and should go barefoot and strive to walk unassisted. You may never desire to run barefoot, but you may kick off your shoes for life.

Use It or Lose It

When it comes to your body, there's one simple principle you have to respect: Use it or lose it. If you don't use your body, well, nature's not so kind. Whether it's a broken arm or hip, your cardiovascular strength, or anything else, if you use it, it gets stronger, and if not, it weakens. If you don't work a muscle, it gets weaker as your body delivers nourishment to muscles that need it more.

As Dr. Henry S. Lodge states in *Younger Next Year*, you can get healthier and fitter at almost any age. If you stimulate the mind and body, it can regenerate at any age. And this doesn't just go for strengthening an arm, hip, or back. This goes for strengthening your mind as well. Use your body by going barefoot, and in this case you will feel the ground and wake up your nervous system, vestibular system, vision and balance, stimulate new brain cell growth, create new maps in your mind—literally, sharpening your mind in the process.

As neuroplastician Dr. Michael Merzenich told me in a recent phone conversation, you're never too old to start, and you can gain back losses, at least when it comes to the mind. No matter what your age, if you start working out, or using your body more, it gets stronger. The human body can wake up—so who cares how many candles are on your next birthday cake?

Dr. Lodge and his coauthor Chris Crowley talk about how we must become full-time athletes once we pass the age of 60. You need to commit to your health in order to stay young, healthy, and fit, or to get back to the fitness you had when you were 60.

Now, I'm not past the age of 60, but having broken my hip, I understand a bit about this philosophy and why you or your grandmother might not be so excited about physical activity. Doctors told me I couldn't, shouldn't, and wouldn't be able to run again. They advised against exercise, rather than more of it.

But this isn't the first time I've heard this warning. Ever since my first serious injury, a broken femur, tibia, and patella (upper and lower leg and knee) at the age of 10, I've been told time after time that if I work out, I'll risk injury and just make things worse. I was also diagnosed with an arthritic knee at the age of 16 and told to back off. And yet by working out, the arthritis, along with every other "condition" or "challenge" has magically gone away. I've proven to be a "medical miracle." But I'm not. I've just committed to working out 6 days a week to recover and build myself stronger.

So the advice for you older readers and for your parents and grandparents is to commit to working out daily, strengthen what you have, challenge yourself, and see yourself get stronger.

Barefoot Benefits for Seniors

In the PBS special, *The Art of Aging, The Limitless Potential of the Brain*, Ryohei Omiya demonstrates you can reverse the effects of aging on the brain starting at any age.

In 2004, Ryohei set the national record in Japan for the 100+ age group in the 100-meter dash. The record still holds today.

However, at a younger age, Ryohei couldn't run. At 85, he suffered a stroke. Four years later, when his wife died, he stopped running and began to show signs of mild dementia.

"He stayed in his room all day. He sort of drowsed with his mouth open. We [Ryohei's family] all just got the feeling … that his health was failing. At the time he leaned on me to walk and he didn't walk far, not even 100 meters. We were afraid he might slip too," shared Hiroki Omiya, Ryohei's daughter-in-law.

In an effort to improve Ryohei's health, Ryohei's family began taking him out to get some exercise. Remarkably, his interest in life returned and at 99, Ryohei began running again.

Exercise for your brain

Until 1998, there was no hard evidence that brain cells known as neurons regenerate—a term called neurogenesis. The accepted assumption was that nerve cells regenerate in all parts of the body except for the brain and spinal cord. We also thought 100,000 neurons (out of 100 billion) died on a daily basis and could never be restored.

Thanks to the work of Dr. Peter Eriksson, a researcher at the Department of Clinical Neuroscience at Sahlgrenska University Hospital in Sweden, we now know that neurons regenerate even in the brains of the elderly. New brain cells are formed whenever we stimulate the brain, and challenging and different stimula help the most.

Hundreds of studies point to the rejuvenating benefits of exercise. Just think, your brain doesn't have to get weaker, but instead can grow stronger.

Going barefoot literally wakes up your mind.

In *The Brain That Changes Itself*, Dr. Norman Doidge writes:

> "If we went barefoot, our brains would receive many different kinds of input as we went over uneven surfaces. Shoes are a relatively flat platform that spreads out the stimuli, and the surfaces we walk on are increasingly artificial and perfectly flat. This leads us to dedifferentiate the [brain] maps for the soles of our feet and limit how touch guides our foot control. Then we may

start to use canes, walkers, or crutches or rely on other senses to steady ourselves. By resorting to these compensations instead of exercising our failing brain systems, we hasten their decline."

When we go barefoot, we wake up a sixth sense of the body that feels and reads the ground. These new sensations create fresh brain cells, neural pathways, and neural nets in our brains—in essence, helping us begin to regain brain function.

Additionally, by learning how to coordinate our bodies and gain balance by going barefoot, we're creating additional neural pathways in our brains and throughout the nervous system in our bodies. In essence, going barefoot is helping us grow stronger minds, wake up our mind-body connection, and rewire our brains.

Feeling the ground for the first time is like learning a foreign language, or playing a new musical instrument. It requires the brain to process information in a novel way, with new dimensions and sensations never perceived before. This dramatically helps stimulate the mind as it forces the mind to relearn how to learn.

Just standing on a cobblestone mat helps begin to rewire the mind. However,

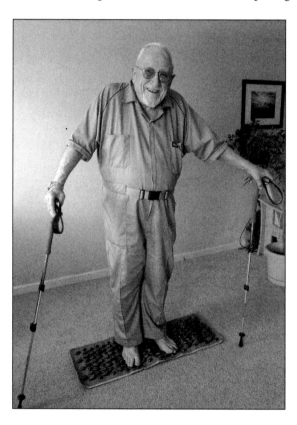

Bill Weber at 91 wakes up his feet on a cobblestone mat. Just weeks later he was out and about, without his walking sticks.

imagine walking or even running barefoot on uneven surfaces and how much that would stimulate your mind. A good barefoot walk on a trail would be like reading a Braille novel with your feet, giving incredible stimulus to help wake up the brain.

Balance

The most important key to fitness in seniors is balance. Why? If you're balanced, you can climb stairs, walk, or even run without the fear of falling and breaking a hip—one of the most serious injuries seniors face.

Going barefoot and feeling the ground is one of the best ways in the world to gain balance. When you're in a shoe, you can't feel the ground, and you're literally walking or running blind without any input as to what's beneath you. Ever tried standing on one foot? Perhaps it wasn't too tough. Now try doing it with your eyes closed. We all tend to teeter pretty quickly with the loss of just this one sense. The difference is as dramatic when going barefoot versus wearing a shoe.

When our feet touch the ground barefoot, we wake up the nerve endings on the bottom of our feet and grow new neural pathways in our brains, which help teach our bodies how to stabilize and get balanced. In essence, we're rewiring our brains for balance and, ultimately, for much more, as new neural nets improve other cognitive skills.

Gaining or regaining balance is not as simple as taking off your shoes. In fact, studies show that if you just get out of your shoes, you'll initially have less balance than before. This makes sense because your muscles are weak and shoe dependent, and you haven't done the mental training to learn to stabilize yourself.

Instead, try this: If you're still quite mobile, an avid walker, or a runner, simply start slowly incorporating barefoot time into your routine. You want to work on waking up nerve endings on the bottom of your feet. Start with a little time standing barefoot. Then begin walking barefoot on a cobblestone mat to wake up the dormant nerve endings. Note, if your mobility is already compromised, seek assistance from a friend, family member, or medical professional depending on your needs.

Once, you're comfortable spending time barefoot, you can start incorporating balance exercises. The next step would be to do one-legged standing exercises. You can begin these by holding onto a wall, a railing, or someone standing next to you. At first, spend a minute or two each day barefoot, just practicing standing on one leg, and then the other. (Order a RunBare Balance Kit at www.RunBare.com.)

Over time, you can progress to a low teeter board, standing at first on the board with both legs at a time, while you hold onto something in front of you. Begin with just a minute or two. Then build up from there—working on the ability to balance hands free.

Jack's Story

A good friend and mentor of mine, Jack Burden, was 81 when he realized he was losing a lot of his strength and locomotion. He began to exercise in a gym. He started working on a treadmill, working up to 3.5 mph. In addition, he worked with weights to strengthen his upper body, and he worked on a BOSU balance trainer to improve his balance, which was deteriorating. On this trainer, which is a round inflated 10-inch-high ball that resembles the top of a ball attached to a platform, he eventually had no problem keeping his balance for 7 minutes or more, some of the time with his eyes closed.

He has not been able to use a cobblestone mat or a teeter board because a painful bunion on his left foot hurts when he's barefoot. He would love to walk or jog barefoot, but short of an operation to correct the problem, it's just too painful. Instead, he bounces and jogs barefoot on a Needak mini trampoline. The trampoline does not provide the grounding he would get going barefoot, but it does greatly improve his balance, strengthens his cells, muscles, bones, major organs, and brain. His lymphatic fluids are forcefully flushed though the lymph nodes and out of the body as well.

At 87, he also hikes in the mountains west of Boulder on trails classified as easy to moderately difficult.

Building strong bones

If you're not weight bearing or stressing your muscles, you lose bone. One of the leading reasons our bones get brittle is because we're not exercising or using our muscles enough. This becomes cyclical too. If you're worried about falling and breaking a hip, you may exercise less or move less in general. With the use-it-or-lose-it principle, if you do less, you lose what you have, in this case bone density, making you more prone to breaking a hip.

As you're working on balance, you can begin building stronger bones. Better balance helps you prevent falling, and staying mobile helps your bones get strong. The two work hand in hand. Not only that, but if your bones are stronger, chances are you can handle a trip or fall without a serious injury. It doesn't matter how many calcium supplements you take, if you don't do weight-bearing exercises, you lose bone density and develop that dreaded brittle-bone disorder called osteoporosis.

According to Dr. Gary Null, author of *Be a Healthy Women*, "Not only is weight training safe, it is important for preventing osteoporosis. As muscles are pulled directly against the bone, with gravity working against it, calcium is driven back into the bones. It also stimulates the manufacture of new bone. This adds up to a decrease in the effects of osteoporosis by 50 to 80 percent." Additionally studies are showing that arthritic joints can regain mobility through exercise.

Going barefoot and gaining stability, coordination, and balance helps you gain the freedom you need to break this cycle. You can regain the bone density you once had, or grow your bones back stronger.

When you're barefoot, you're stimulating muscles, tendons, ligaments, and ultimately the bones found in feet, legs, and hips. Since you're relying on your feet, legs, and stabilizing muscles to give you balance, rather than your shoes, you are working and stimulating more muscle and bones throughout your entire body, and in particular the muscles and bones of the hip.

Doing balance exercises barefoot, walking barefoot, or yes, jogging barefoot, all can help you keep the bones you have, grow them stronger, and help prevent that dreaded hip-breaking fall to begin with.

FOOT NOTE

While I advocate cross-training activities such as swimming and cycling to supplement running and walking, we believe weight-bearing exercises, such as running and walking, are the best for building bone density, muscle strength, balance, and overall fitness. In a 2008 study published in *Metabolism*, researchers measured bone mineral density in 43 competitive male cyclists and runners ages 20 to 59. Their findings found that compared to runners, cyclists had significantly lower bone mineral density of the whole body. Compared to 19 percent of runners, 63 percent of the cyclists had osteopenia (precursor to osteoporosis) of the spine or hip, and cyclists were 7 times more likely to have osteopenia of the spine than the runners.

Gaining cardiovascular strength

Running is what keeps us alive and keeps us healthy. Dr. Daniel Lieberman, an evolutionary biologist from Harvard cautions, "Not running is the most harmful thing we can do to our bodies."

No matter our age, if we keep our heart and lungs healthy, it increases the quality of our lives. This is why authors Lodge and Crowley advocate becoming a full-time athlete—working out 6 days a week, especially after 60. If you can keep running, jogging, or doing other aerobic activities, you greatly increase the quality of your life in almost every respect. This is largely due to the endorphins and other chemicals released in the brain during cardiovascular workouts. These natural happy drugs improve mood, possess anti-inflammatory qualities, boost the immune system, and much more.

Running and aerobic exercise has been shown to greatly reduce symptoms of tension, anxiety, and depression. It strengthens the heart and lungs, increases blood flow, and helps the body eliminate toxins (all which help you feel better).

Cardio exercises also serve to keep body fat and obesity down. This can have a significant effect on the health of seniors, as keeping weight off of the joints allows you to continue to be active and gain mobility and fitness, even if frail or arthritic.

When we go barefoot and strengthen our feet and legs, aerobic exercise becomes far more available to us. Now this can be barefoot running or brisk walking, both great ways to build strength and balance, or simply using our barefoot time to do more traditional exercises in the gym as well.

Stronger core

When you go without shoes, you use your core (your stomach and back muscles) to keep you balanced. This has particular importance for freedom, mobility, and remaining pain-free as a senior. Many seniors suffer from back pain, which was often traced back to an earlier injury or trauma, and then exacerbated by inactivity, an unhealthy lifestyle, deteriorating posture, and a weak back.

When you strengthen your core, you help protect and strengthen your back, take your guarded muscles out of spasm, and make them more pain-free. This is the theory behind the practice of Pilates. Founder Joseph Pilates was able to keep his back strong and healthy well into his 80s. A strong core improves posture and helps your back be more mobile, flexible, strong, and pain-free. This helps seniors in all daily activities.

Grounding effect

Touching the ground barefoot doesn't just feel good; it is good for you. It helps you drain off an excess electrical charge you're carrying on your skin and sync you with the vibrational frequency of the earth. As studies have shown, this has far-reaching health benefits, from reduced inflammation, reduced effects of arthritis, fights off free radicals, which damage and age our cells, bolsters the immune system, and creates even greater natural cancer-fighting agents in our body. That, coupled with the anti-anxiety and anti-depression effects, makes getting grounded almost a must as part of staying healthy at any age and as you age.

Reflexology

Reflexology is the practice of massaging or relieving tension, improving circulation, and helping return the natural function to all parts of the body by stimulating pressure points or zones on the hands, feet, or ears, but in particular, in the feet.

When you go barefoot, you stimulate all of the reflex points on the bottom of your feet, helping reduce tension, improve body function, reduce inflammation, and much more. Studies are suggesting reflexology not only strengthens your immune system, but fights cancer.

In a pilot study, Oregon Research Institute scientists engaged men and women aged 60 to 88 in a cobblestone mat walking activity for 8 weeks. At the end of the trial, the walking participants experienced improvements in psychophysical well-being, reductions in daily sleepiness and pain, significant improvement in perceptions of control over falls, and reduced blood pressure—a classic reflexology response.

Footwear for Seniors

I recommend low footwear with flexible soles and no high heels. If the flexible sole is too much, begin with a hard sole, but the key is to be low to the ground. Again you want a wide toe box to allow the toes to wake up and to move.

Studies are showing if you can get an uneven or bumpy foot bed inside of your shoe, you can wake up nerve endings too. While such a foot bed would not get you closer to the ground (therefore not aiding with stability), it may be a way to safely wake up nerve endings in your feet.

Wake Up Your Feet

It's never too late to go barefoot, and the health benefits can literally change your life. From helping give you greater balance, strength, mobility, and freedom, to better cognitive functions, a potentially stronger immune system and more, the benefits of going barefoot as a senior are too great to be ignored.

Start slowly, even a little barefoot walking, or standing next to a beam can help to begin. Gradually increase your distance and begin doing balance exercises. Over time you'll awaken the nerves on the bottom of your feet. You'll strengthen your feet and stabilizing muscles. You'll gain bone density, joint mobility, and more.

Overall, going barefoot gives you greater health and freedom. Who says you have to sit around or stay in shoes as you age? Instead, why not get younger, this year, next year, and the ones thereafter. Give it a chance! Hop out of your shoes, wake up those feet, and have fun.

PART V

If You Really Must Wear Something on Your Feet

It took the whole of Creation to produce my foot, my each feather: Now I hold Creation in my foot.

—Hawk Roosting

16

Minimalist Shoes and Other Essential Gear

Some women have a weakness for shoes. I can go barefoot if necessary. I have a weakness for books.

—Oprah Winfrey

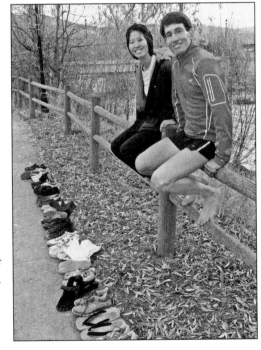

"We're not against shoes, just against bad shoes that will hurt you." The authors test shoes in Steamboat Springs, Colorado.

admit it. I like shoes. They can be filled with style and fun. So I'm not against shoes. I'm just against bad shoes that hurt our feet and don't let us move naturally or feel the ground. Shoes have their purpose. For either necessity or social norms and to get served in restaurants, you too may need a new shoe now and again.

In simplest terms, minimalist footwear is footwear that lets your foot do the work and doesn't impede the natural gait or stride that barefoot running promotes. More natural shoes tend to be much lighter, lower, flatter, wider, and more flexible while far less supportive, restrictive, or controlling than the majority of shoes out there today.

Personally, I like to go barefoot all the time. But there's a time and place for footwear. When I'm heading to the grocery or a restaurant, I'm in footwear. If I've toasted my pads and want another run, I'm in footwear; and if I'm heading out for a snowy, icy run, I may be in footwear.

For the Times You Must Wear Shoes

Here are more times and places you may choose to go shod:

- **Transitioning to barefoot running.** Even after your first few months, you may not be ready for a zero-arch shoe. Consider using shoes with incrementally less of an arch to wean yourself into them. Think of arch support as training wheels. As your feet grow stronger, you'll need shoes less and less until you remove them entirely.

  I strongly recommend going unshod for training (every other day) for your first 2 to 3 months. This lets your skin be your guide and safely builds foot strength fast. In between your barefoot runs use your current shoes, insoles, or orthotics as recovery aids.

- **For challenging terrain.** Even for the most experienced barefoot runner, some surfaces such as gravel, snow and ice, melting hot pavement, or perhaps chip and seal roads, may require shoes. If the going may get tough, bring your shoes along, they may come in handy.

To prevent infections.

- If you're running in a third-world country where parasites abound, or anywhere sanitation, standing water, or sewage may be a problem, and especially if you have a cut or an open wound, wear your shoes.

- **As training tools**

  o **For mileage.** Foot padding is like muscle: the more you challenge it, the more it needs rest to grow back stronger. After your first few months, if you're careful, you can run shod in between barefoot days while allowing your pads to recover.

o **For speed.** Though many of the faster runners train barefoot, almost all still race in shoes. Specificity is the name of the game. If you'll be racing in shoes, you'll need some training in shoes. Consider alternating between shod and unshod runs, making sure at least half of your speed work is done in shoes.

o **After workouts.** Speed tears up pads. When I'm out for a tempo run or track repeats, I bring my shoes along. Once the pads are toasty, I throw on my shoes and slowly jog home.

o **For strength.** Different shoes work your feet in different ways. For instance, the Newton takes you off the ground and far from your heels. Alternating between a model or two of minimalist shoes—along with barefoot training—helps you stretch, strengthen, and stress different ligaments, tendons, and muscle groups to build the strongest feet you can. Just remember, almost all shoes eliminate awareness. If you train in a shoe, focus on landing extra light with proper form.

• **For racing.** Unless you have feet of steel or run the smoothest of courses, initially you'll be faster racing in a shoe. Racing in minimalist footwear protects your feet from road debris and trashing your pads at speed. Wear the least shoe you can, stay on your forefoot, and focus on a short stride.

In public.

• Unless you're trying to make a statement, bring footwear along for grocery stores, restaurants, or places people may balk. Personally, I love walking barefoot in our local, stone-tiled mall, but when it comes to food-related stores, I'm always in a shoe. My choice for public footwear is Japanese Tatami mat bamboo sandals, which let my feet breathe and toes spread and rest upon a more natural surface.

• **At work.** Consider those flexible shoes that are easy to kick off under your desk if you sit at work. Shoe companies such as Vivo Barefoot and Earth footwear make casual minimalist shoes that may be work-appropriate.

• **At school.** While studies show children are best left unshod, good luck with your school administrators or your child's PE teacher. Find good natural footwear for class (Feelmax accommodates kids sizes) and more protective shoes for field activities where spiked shoes are involved.

If you have a foot pathology.

- Whether nature or nurture, some feet may never fully take to barefoot running (perhaps too many years in shoes, or surgery). However, barefoot walking and feeling the ground is still fantastic for your health. If your feet have seen extra woes, wake them extra slowly both in and out of shoes. Focus on barefoot walking rather than running, more recovery time, and a slower transition to natural, less supportive shoes.

Don't Trust Your Shoe Salesman

It's not their fault nor are they intentionally overlooking your best interests, but the average shoe salesman is indoctrinated by a constant barrage of footwear propaganda, "product education," and marketing hype each year. They want to help, but may not know the best solutions.

Here's false propaganda to watch out for:

- Pronation (or rolling the foot downward and inward) is bad, and if you pronate you *must* use motion control or stability shoes. *Not true, particularly over time.* You may just need to *strengthen* your foot.

- If you get sore knees, you need more cushioning. *False.* Cushioning makes you hit harder and causes sore knees.

- Materials in most shoes compress so fast they lose their cushioning almost overnight. *Not true.* You want to feel the ground. Even with hundreds of miles on your shoes, they're likely still too cushioned.

- Shoes must be replaced every 300 to 400 miles. *False.* The older the shoe, the more naturally your foot moves and feels the ground, and the less likely you'll suffer an injury. So dig out those comfortable old soles and put 'em back on.

- Racing flats don't last. *False.* While there's less cushion, the shoe still lasts for hundreds of miles.

- Shoe store video analysis reveals all. I wish this were true but it depends on the analyst and the test. For instance, standing or walking on a force plate reveals little or nothing as your dynamics completely change for running. Additionally, running on a treadmill, even barefoot, rarely reveals more than just a weak foot. Almost every bare foot reveals pronation; if the foot's weak, it needs strengthening. And if it's strong, the foot pronates to store and return energy. When you're strong, pronation's good. Haile Gebrselassie shows massive pronation as he loads the foot and springs back. Yet a treadmill test would put him in a heavy motion control shoe.

- A properly fitting shoe cures all. If only this were the case, but it's much more than fit. Today's shoes have high heels, toes, heavy cushioning and more. Even if your foot fit the shoe well, if it doesn't meet much of the following parameters, it's still likely to hurt you.

- Running shoes should fit snug. *False.* I fell for this one for years and opted for narrower and narrower shoes until I wound up in a women's AA width shoe. Feet adapt to the size of their environment. A small, narrow shoe creates a small, narrow foot. Additionally, snug shoes don't allow your feet to expand when they contact the ground, putting more force on a smaller area of the foot while decreasing stability. If your toes can't spread, your foot is in trouble. Fortunately, my feet have returned to a more natural, wider width.

- Your arch height determines the amount of support you need. *False.* Many people ask, "What shoe is good for a high or low arch?" However, the better question to ask is, "How much support do I need for a weak or strong arch?" Just because someone has a high arch, it does not mean you give them a big arch support. When you run barefoot, your arches naturally get stronger and taller—and you need less arch support. There's no right or wrong arch height, or one height that needs support more than another. It's arch strength that needs to be taken into account.

Natural footwear

No shoe is perfect, and until it is, barefoot may be best. According to Dr. William Rossi, a podiatrist with 8 books on footwear and over 400 published articles, there's no way to have a natural gait or stride when in a shoe. He defines natural as being the pure or ideal, and normal as being the closest to the norm. For instance, he says the common cold may be normal, but it isn't natural and isn't healthy. He makes this astute observation:

It took four million years to develop our unique human foot and our consequent distinctive form of gait, a remarkable feat of bioengineering. Yet, in only a few thousand years, and with one carelessly designed instrument, our shoes, we have warped the pure anatomical form of human gait, obstructing its engineering efficiency, afflicting it with strains and stresses and denying it its natural grace of form and ease of movement head to foot. We have converted a beautiful thoroughbred into a plodding plowhorse.

Michael's Checklist for Selecting a Minimalist Shoe

The goal of minimalist or natural footwear is to allow you the most natural stride possible. To do so, we must throw out much of the junk designed into shoes today such as elevated heels, arches, stability, motion control, curved toes (called toe-spring) and much more.

No shoe is perfect, but some are far better than others. With new shoes coming on the market almost daily, use this guide to weigh the plusses and minuses of your selection.

☐ **Light weight.** Any weight on your foot changes the dynamic of the stride, and the heavier the shoe, the more your stride changes. Weight can cause your heel to drop first, or put undue stress and strain on the shins, which were never designed to carry weight in the first place. A good minimalist shoe is exceptionally lightweight, no more than 6 to 8 ounces (170–227 grams) or less per shoe. Unfortunately, this takes many shoes out of the running that claim to give you a more natural stride.

●°°°₀ FOOT NOTE

Even at 100 strides a minute, in a pair of 8-ounce shoes, you're lifting a pound per stride, 100 pounds a minute, or 3 tons an hour. Double the weight of the shoe for a supportive trainer, and you're carrying 6 tons of weight on your feet and legs per hour. That's the weight of a good-sized elephant. No wonder joints crumble!

☐ **Low to the ground.** The number one acute running injury is ankle sprains, and there's no better way to lose stability than being high up off the ground such as in a well-cushioned shoe. You gain greater stability and feel of the ground as you get lower. Consider shoes that are ideally a centimeter off the ground or less.

☐ **No heel lift.** Even if the shoe is close to the ground, if it's not flat, it's trouble. The trend in running shoes is higher heels, which unfortunately rotates your pelvis and shifts your weight unnaturally forward. This forces you to change the angle of your ankles, knees, hips, back, shoulders, and neck leading to soreness and serious overuse injuries over time. Ideally, consider shoes with less than 2 to 4 mm discrepancy between heel height and toe. Even a centimeter's difference substantially affects your stride economy and safety.

☐ **Little or no toe-spring.** When barefoot, your toes sit flat on the ground and grab for propulsion. But shoes curve the front of the foot up eliminating the use of your toes. Footwear manufacturers think this makes it easier to run, but since 18 out of 19 muscles and tendons of the foot connect to your toes, this construction weakens your entire foot and radically changes the dynamics of your stride. Consider shoes with little or no toe-spring. True flats or shoes without a curve in front are best for a more natural stride, stronger healthier feet, and better stability and propulsion.

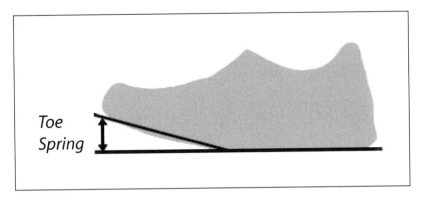

Steer clear of toe-spring. With 18 of 19 muscles and tendons of the feet connecting to your toes, strong toes mean strong feet. Yet shoes that curve upward eliminate the use of your toes, weakening feet, changing stride, and making you unstable.

☐ **Wide toe box.** Stay clear of narrow shoes, even if they meet all other criteria. Your foot naturally expands with each stride, both as a spring, and for stability. Many minimalist shoes such as cross-country racing flats and other track shoes do not let your feet expand. This forces more weight on a smaller area, which leads to overuse injuries such as tendonitis and stress fractures, and also creates a very unstable platform on which to land. Women, you may want to consider the men's version of your favorite shoe to get the room you need in the forefoot.

☐ **No arch support.** Your foot can't move naturally if the arch is propped up. Ideally, you want zero support for your arch. Any more than that keeps your arch weak. However, if you've been locked in a traditional shoe for years, you may want to wean off slowly, at least in between barefoot workouts. Go with much less arch support than the shoe salesman recommends. If it's truly holding your foot in place, you've got far too much support. (A key point: As your feet get strong, even minimal arch support can become a true danger. Not only will it change your stride and prevent your foot from absorbing shock naturally, but if your feet are strong enough to support you on your own, that little arch support will cause your feet to roll to the outside or suppinate. Suppination can cause serious IT band problems, and knee, hip, and particularly, ankle and shin problems. If you're doing just fine barefoot, you'll need a shoe without arch support, or your foot and leg will be rolled to the outside.)

- **Avoid narrow lasts.** Often, though not always, a shoe manufacturer tries to throw an arch or arch support into a lightweight shoe or racing flat without hardened plastic or molding by making the last narrow in the middle—thus making the tight, narrow mid-section of the shoe support your arch. This is just another way to make an arch support, which you want little or none of.

- **No motion control.** The majority of shoes today are designed to move your foot from one place to another through your stride. This motion completely negates the foot's desire to naturally go where it wants, and that's even if the shoe was designed for forefoot striking. Most shoes are made to control your foot for a heel strike. Forcing your foot to move in any one plane or direction of travel creates a conflict between the foot's desire to go one way and the shoe's desire to go another—thereby creating injury. Avoid shoes with strong groves or channels along the sole that lock your foot in place.

- **Avoid multiple sole patterns and materials.** Shoe manufacturers often vary the density or type of foam and rubber on their soles along with the tread to make your foot move or roll in a particular direction. This is also a means of motion control. You want one material on the bottom, so your foot can choose where it goes, rather than being dictated by the softness or firmness of the rubber on the sole.

- **Look for a straight-axis shoe.** Shoes without in-flare or "banana-nosed" shoes are still hard to come by. Shoes are built on a "last" or sole, and then material is wrapped around them. While our feet are built on a straight axis, the majority of shoes are still built with the toes curving toward the insides of our feet, called in-flare. This is why we wear out the tops of our shoes first and end up deforming our shoes to the outside. It's always why we end up with curved toes after the age of 6, according to Dr. Rossi. Our feet and toes want to move one way, and our shoes forces them another. This doesn't just do cosmetic damage as the toes are connected to nearly every ligament and tendon of the foot. Look for a shoe that lets your foot stay as straight as possible on the inside.

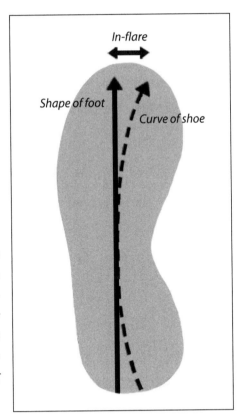

Beware of in-flare. While feet are nearly straight, modern running shoes curve like a banana. This curve deforms your feet, crams your toes, wreaks havoc on your stride, and prevents your feet from moving and absorbing shock naturally.

□ **Beware of shoe concavity.** The majority of footbeds today are also concave in the forefoot. This was done for style (to make the foot appear slimmer) 80 years ago and continued for tradition through today. Unfortunately, as the insole breaks down further, it produces a deeper cavity or recess for the forefoot. This creates several key problems. First, it contributes to a condition called the fallen metatarsal arch—a very painful condition. Second, since the forefoot is no longer flush with the ground, the toes are locked out of grabbing (just as with toe-spring), and the metatarsals can't act as tiny fulcrums or levers. This radically changes your stride and force dynamics. In other words, this small change made for style in footwear can lead to injuries throughout your entire body.

□ **Look for a flexible sole.** Out of a shoe your toes naturally flex 54 degrees at the ball of the foot, but in a shoe, they flex 30 to 80 percent less, according to Dr. Rossi. The more flexible the sole, the more your foot flexes naturally and feels the ground. This aids with foot strength, stability, circulation, recovery, and flexibility. However, such flexibility can be detrimental, particularly in the beginning, on rocky terrain. Work into more flexible soles over time as your feet gain strength, flexibility, and padding.

If not, you're looking at overuse injuries or because rocks are felt straight through the shoe, even an acute injury such as a fractured metatarsal, from slamming your foot into a rock. In general, the more flexible the sole, the better you'll feel the ground, mitigate shock, and strengthen your feet.

You can test the flexibility of a shoe, not by folding it in half, but by putting your hand in the shoe up to where the ball of your foot would be, then with your other hand, flex the toes or forefoot of the shoe. If there's resistance, your foot will have to work harder with each and every step, which can greatly throw off your balance.

☐ **Stay away from heavy cushioning.** Recently someone told me, "It's the most comfortable shoe I've ever run in." However, the shoe he spoke of was a heavily cushioned clunker. Instead of protecting his feet, he was likely hurting himself. Cushioned comfort's not the key; a plush luxury automobile might feel great on the highway, but be deadly on the racetrack. Cushioning reduces your ability to feel the ground, causing you to strike harder. It also makes your foot squirm and reduces stability. This can lead to overuse injuries throughout your feet, ankles, knees, and elsewhere (particularly your sensitive IT bands, which were never designed to stabilize a squirmy leg) and can lead to a trip or fall (and subsequent sprained ankle or worse). You'd never catch a baseball with a boxing glove, so why would you try to run while wearing one? Get the least cushioning you can.

◉°°°₀ FOOT NOTE

"Ironically, the closest we have ever come to an 'ideal' shoe was the original lightweight, soft-sole, heel-less, simple moccasin, which dates back more than 14,000 years. It consisted of a piece of crudely tanned but soft leather wrapped around the foot and held on with rawhide thongs. Presto! Custom fit, perfect in biomechanical function, and no encumbrances to the foot or gait."

—Dr. William Rossi

☐ **Make sure they're breathable.** Feet sweat, and hot feet sweat profusely. As barefoot runners, foot sweat is death. Not only does it allow fungus and molds to quickly set up shop, but soaks your pads and wears away your skin. Additionally, foot odor doesn't exist in nature—it only exists in a shoe. Hot stinky shoes are a terrible way to maintain the toughened skin you've worked so hard to build. Hot feet also swell, which can lead to a whole host of health problems. According to podiatrist Dr. Michael Nirenberg, "Swelling or edema of feet can lead to poor perfusion of blood to the tissues, constriction, varicose veins, joint stiffness, diminished function, and symptoms of pain, heaviness, cramping, and restlessness." Your foot can slide in sweaty shoes and contribute to a lack of stability and control. In the summer, get a light-colored shoe. You'd never go out in black clothing in the summer, so why would you wear black shoes?

- **Slip on.** Can the shoes slide on and off easily or fold up for easy transport? The more convenient your shoes, the more you'll use them when the going gets tough, and stow them away when things ease up. Though not essential, a slip-on, slip-off shoe, or one without a lace can make things far easier and convenient. Additionally, laces tend to bind, a great lace-free shoe may help your foot move and feel more naturally.

- **Green.** Look for eco-friendly shoes that are made with recycled materials or locally made whenever possible and always vote with your dollars. Also consider supporting the "little guys" too. The smaller, less-conventional shoe manufacturers need our support and have more on the line. They tend to be the most innovative, receptive to new ideas, and are likely to drive future trends.

How to Wear Minimalist Footwear

Maybe it's ironic because I am a barefoot running coach, but I recommend owning at least a couple different pairs of minimalist footwear if possible: one pair that really lets you feel the ground, and another that's a bit stiffer and potentially has just a bit of an arch for recovery. In this manner, if the skin of your feet is tired from barefoot running, you can still get out, as long as you are careful.

Use shoes as training and recovery tools, but watch your fatigue levels. Since your skin should be your guide, if you feel like taking the day off, don't try to nurse yourself along in a shoe. But if your feet are only mildly fatigued, and you've been building gradually, consider heading out slowly in a slightly more supportive and protective shoe.

If your feet aren't fatigued, or if you can't go barefoot because of the cold, choose a shoe in which you can fully feel the ground. For instance, after a really hard workout, it's possible I'll let my feet recover while wearing my Asics Piranhas or Adidas Adizero PRs. And if my feet feel nice and loose, but I've toasted my pads a bit, or it's well below freezing, I'll head out in my Sockwas or neoprene moccasins.

Shoes can be important training tools—and necessary in some climates. Just try not to stick to any one particular shoe day after day. Rotate through several pairs during a week if possible to work your feet in different ways or allow them to recover.

Few barefoot runners will be barefoot 100 percent of the time. Personally, I'm about 90 percent barefoot in the warmer months, and perhaps 50 percent barefoot through the winter. No matter how much or little you wear shoes, consider the following.

To sock or not to sock?

I avoid socks if at all possible. Once you've been going barefoot, your feet generate much more heat than traditionally shod feet. And even if you haven't been going barefoot, your feet have to work more in minimalist footwear, so you tend to pump more warm blood to the feet, rather than less. Unless it's too cold, I'd recommend staying out of socks to keep your feet closer to the ground, to keep your feet from sliding around (which could create a whole host of problems and challenges), and to keep your feet from getting hot, wet, and sweaty. As barefoot runners, we abhor moisture, and even in the most wickable socks, this is hard to avoid.

Now there is one consideration for socks: the cold. If it's cold and your feet can't get warm, then by all means, put on some socks. Try to find the thinnest socks that work for you. Personally, if I'm wearing my racing flats, I like some lycra, scuba-type socks called Hotskins by Henderson Aquatics because they're less than 2 mm thick (as long as my feet won't slide too much). But I'm typically in my neoprene moccasins, and if that's the case and it's really cold (below zero) I'll be in the thinnest Smartwool hiking or running sock I can get. (I like Smartwool over synthetics because it'll keep my feet warm, even if my feet get wet. This can be a lifesaver!)

Get a loose sock. Too tight socks constrict blood flow and cool off the foot. I'm careful once I'm wearing socks, because I can't feel the ground as well (and I may strike the ground too hard), move around differently in my moccasins, my stride changes, and I'm not nearly as stable as being barefoot in a shoe. Squishy wintertime socks are often an invitation to an overuse injury.

How about insoles, orthotics, and footbeds?

In short, for some people there is a time and a place for insoles and orthotics, particularly if there is a true foot pathology or past foot surgery. For those who wear them and are getting into barefoot running, insoles may be an excellent recovery tool or device to wear in between your barefoot runs as you gradually build up your feet.

As for traditional footbeds you find in all but the most minimalist shoes or racing flats, I'd recommend removing them if at all possible. Footbeds typically add 2 mm or more (I've seen 4 mm in a few shoes) to the height of your foot in an effort to give you extra cushioning or support—two things you're trying to avoid. In other words, they raise you up in the shoe and cushion you, making you less stable, and making it harder to feel the ground.

Footbeds may also give you arch support, which you don't want or likely don't need. So unless you need the support (or are weaning your way off them), pull the insoles out of your shoes, unless you have to tear your shoes apart to do so.

Keeping your feet dry

If you're in a shoe, chances are your feet are going to get wet. As long as your feet don't slide around too much, and you can keep your shoes clean and fungal-free (if they're smelling even a little, it's far beyond time to wash them), the wet feet aren't too much of a problem.

I recommend using climbing chalk or synthetic chalk after your runs to dry off your feet and pads quickly. Of course, first hit the shower, then apply the chalk.

Laces

While they may be a necessary evil, I'm not a big fan of shoelaces. I don't like how they unevenly distribute force or bind our feet. Many of us have stories or know of other runners who've hurt their feet by running or racing with laces bound too tight.

If you're going to lace up, I recommend keeping them loose, but not quite to the point where your feet slide around. Consider switching to a wide flat lace that will stay in place (as long as they don't get twisted) and won't dig into your foot. Better yet, look for shoes with alternate binding systems (such as Velcro or a drawstring) or no laces at all.

Sizing

In so many things when it comes to barefoot running, good is bad and wrong is right. The same can most certainly be said for sizing. No longer do you want a snug, tight-fitting shoe. Instead, you want something roomy, which allows your toes to spread.

Especially for women, whose shoes tend to be incredibly snug in the front, you want to get a shoe that's wide enough for completely unencumbered movement of the toes. This may mean choosing the men's model in the correct size, or even bumping up a half to a full size to accommodate your toes.

Typically, feet change size when you go barefoot as well, on average, one half to a full shoe size as your feet get stronger and gain their more natural shape. Make sure you choose a shoe that allows your toes to curl as well as spread, and if you're looking at a glove-like shoe like the Vibram FiveFingers, choose one that's not too tight across the instep and allows your toes to lift up as well as curl down.

Dangers

Although we don't want to belabor the point, the biggest challenge of minimalist foot-wear is that you can't feel the ground or let your skin be your guide. While running in minimalist shoes, you may feel free, fast, and light for the first time in your life, yet you may ask far too much of your feet, too soon. This can result in a whole host of overuse injuries, which is why we recommend going barefoot first and then going to minimalist shoes later, or using a gentle combination of both.

When it comes to minimalist shoes, it's too easy to be the hare, but when transitioning into barefoot running, the tortoise always wins the race.

All but the most minimal of footwear becomes a road hazard once you get good at barefoot running. You'll need to choose your shoes carefully and watch how you do. Shoes you once thought wide enough, or flat enough, just won't do anymore. Stay aware of your body. It's the best way to prevent problems, which can come on quickly if you're no longer used to traditional shoes.

In any shoe, there are dangers of improper fit. This can be even more of a challenge in minimalist footwear, because now your foot must do the majority of the work. This means an ill-fitting shoe could easily overwork or cook the foot, creating an acute overuse injury, in a very short period of time.

Minor tweaks, pains, and discomforts may be a sign of a future overuse injury anywhere in the leg, not just in the foot. So if the shoe feels too tight, doesn't let your toes move, or doesn't let you use the same stride as if you're barefoot, then no matter how much you like them, or how cool they look, they're not the shoe for you.

Inspirational Footwear

Running barefoot through a muddy puddle can be the best experience in the world. A thin coat of mud forms on the bottom of your feet that acts as a barrier or amazing protection against sharp stones and other challenging elements. I often wish we could just dip our feet into something, let it harden and dry, and then away we go.

To this end, other sports may offer some helpful footwear solutions.

- Martial arts or kung fu shoes, such as those worn by Jackie Chan, in karate classes or at Tai Chi sessions are quite flexible and allow your feet to move freely and feel the ground.

- Wrestling shoes, if you can find any wide enough, are even thinner and amazingly flexible.

- Dancing shoes such as ballet slippers (flats, not toe shoes), if wide enough, offer just enough minimal protection against the ground, while allowing your feet to move naturally.

- Jazz shoes got me through high school. It turns out that I wore jazz shoes to high school when we had a dress code that didn't allow sneakers. I needed to run at least a mile each way with a loaded backpack, so I sought out the most "sneaker-like" shoe I could find. I ended up with Capezio jazz shoes (without a raised heel), which I replaced year after year but used for countless mile after mile. I didn't realize it at the time but they were helping build up foot strength, while at the same time keeping me low, stable, and letting me feel the ground.

- Modern dancers often wear minimal protection on their feet. If you've ever watched modern dance, you'll swear the dancers are barefoot. And for the most part, they are. But with all those twists, turns, jumps, and more on hard parquet floors, they often want something to protect the soles of their feet. Their answer? Tiny leather or synthetic foot pads with the look and feel of being barefoot. These pads are some of the most creative things out there. They cover just the ball of your foot, and nowhere else.

Footwear Review

My original intention was to review all minimalist shoes I could find in this section. But when I started reviewing shoes, I thought I'd find perhaps 10 or 20 pairs of interest. Not so. Dozens started appearing, and I knew a new footwear revolution had begun.

◐°°°。 FOOT NOTE

Online Shoe Reviews

Please go to our Web site at www.RunBare.com and access the Minimalist Shoe Review section. We will continually update the models and our thoughts about them. We'll look at new shoes, old shoes, and be your guide before you step into the shoe department so you can be aware and prepared.

Unless you're barefoot 100 percent of the time—and if so, how do you deal with supermarkets and restaurants?—then you need shoes sometimes. The question is what kind of shoe.

Here are 7 main categories of shoes for you to consider. Of course, every barefoot runner or walker is at his or her own unique place on the spectrum from fully barefoot to needing full support, so judge accordingly.

I discuss the following general categories of shoes in order roughly of most rigid and least barefoot-like to nearly bare. I haven't written about traditional footwear, but realize that modestly supportive shoes (or shoes with a mild arch) may give your feet the rest they need to recover in between barefoot or nearly-barefoot workouts.

1. **Newtons and other toe-running shoes.** I love the concept behind the original Newtons, getting you up and off your heel. I just wish they'd bring you closer to the ground, rather than farther away from it, and wish the lugs were farther forward (as they stand it's more of a midfoot shoe than a true toe-runner's shoe). I think Newtons have their purpose as a training tool, though not as an everyday runner. However, I applaud their efforts as one of a growing group of shoes coming out to help get you off the heel.

Shoes that get you off the heel may help you break old habits. Look for shoes that are light, low, and without extra cushion. Additionally, make sure they don't lock you into a particular stride where your foot can't land on the forefoot where it wants to and move or spring naturally. Some shoes are constraining in this area. You don't want to be locked in a position, even a good one. Injuries often arise when there's a conflict between where your foot wants to go and where your shoe directs it to go.

2. **Tri shoes.** Marketed toward triathletes, tri shoes tend to be fairly light-weight, often slip on quickly, and are better ventilated than traditional running shoes. Tri shoes are distinguished from true racing flats because they're a bit heavier with a higher heel. Yet some of them, such as the K-Swiss, are getting very close to a racing flat. They all tend to have a bit too much of a raised heel. Look for shoes with the least heel possible. Most of them still have a curled up toe (toe-spring) as well, so look for models with the least toe-spring. I like that they're getting lighter and slide on and off quickly. This is ideal for barefoot running when you want to bring your shoes along.

3. **Nike Frees and Free Flexing Shoes.** I love shoes that let your feet flex because it helps you land more naturally and stay more injury-free. Nike Frees are a step in the right direction, I just wish they made it easier to get off the heels and run with a forefoot strike. I'm hopeful this will soon change as similar models by other brands are coming out all the time.

4. **Racing Flats.** I must admit, if I'm going fast in a shoe, these are my shoes of choice—no matter what the distance. My favorite? The Asics Piranha. True flats have little or no toe-spring and do not have a raised heel, making it easier to run on your forefoot and keep you closer to the ground. Each season shoe manufacturers debut more and more new flats. While your regular running-shoe store might not stock many flats, often you can find the best selection at a store that stocks shoes for track and cross-country racers—or online.

5. Vibram FiveFingers and other Glove-like Shoes. Vibrams are just plain different and fun. With individual slots for each of your toes, they let your toes spread and move more freely and let you run with a far more natural style. I'd like them to go further to get even thinner, lighter, and with less binding or restriction between the toes. I think their new Bikila and future models to follow go a definite step in this direction.

The biggest challenge with the FiveFingers is that you still don't feel the ground nearly as much as you do when barefoot, so it's easy to overdo it. Also, some of their models, such as the KSO Trek have built in modest arch support. Now this is not necessarily a bad thing, particularly for a transition shoe, but it is something to watch for.

I can't wait to see what Vibram does next, and what the competition does; yes, expect to see more FiveFingered–type shoes in the marketplace. Remember this, fit is most important. These shoes don't work for everyone. If they bind your toes, prevent free movement (up or down of the toes), or twist or cock your feet when running, then no matter how cool or "in" they seem to be, they may not be for you.

6. Moccasins and Moccasin-like shoes. To me, for the winter, nothing beats my neoprene moccasins, which are really a cycling bootie with an insulated insole. And for walking year-round, a moccasin gives you the closest to barefoot feel of any footwear. However, true leather-made moccasins wear out very quickly unless you use a double-soled version, but then these too will inhibit full proprioception of the ground.

Custom moccasins are also quite costly, particularly given their wear. Other alternatives are Feelmax, which give you a true moccasin-like feel and, with only a 1 mm Kevlar bottom, let you sense the ground beneath you. Feelmax are a great shoe, but because you'll feel everything, they are not a suitable everyday runner until you've built into daily barefoot or near-barefoot runs.

7. Beach socks. Sockwa Beach socks were originally designed for use on the beach. They let your feet move freely and give you the bare minimum of protection for your feet. These can be a smart choice if you're a near full-time barefooter, but just need a bit of protection from the elements. They're just about as close as you can get to barefoot, without being fully barefoot. I love my Beach Sockwas, though you'll wear through them quickly on the roads. Fortunately, they cost a mere fraction of the cost of traditional running shoes.

Honorable mention: Sometimes the best minimalist shoes can be found in dance shoe stores. Modern dance is a version of dance that's performed barefoot or nearly barefoot. In the near-barefoot category, dancers often wear a flesh-colored leather pad (often called a foot thong or dance paws—some actually shaped like a thong) over the ball of the foot to protect the skin from being torn during repeated spins on hardwood floors. There's nothing under the toes, and the leather sole is typically only a millimeter thick, just enough protection to prevent your pads from getting beaten up. These small measures of foot protection allow your toes to fully grab and feel the ground.

I like the Ellis Bella foot thongs. You can find different shapes and sizes that fit your feet best. Many dancers prefer the Capezio Sandasol for its sandal-like look and feel (as it wraps around your heel like a sandal) and at a mere ounce or two, you barely notice you're wearing them.

Think outside the shoe box

As the minimalist trend takes hold, lots of current shoe designs may go by the wayside. That could be challenging for companies unwilling or not eager to change.

We believe that new shoe ideas are going to come from everywhere in the future. From people tinkering in their garages, from insole stores who see a better way and begin to design new things themselves, and from shoe manufacturers—the big boys and the small innovators—who are willing to take a chance and change, and from every place in between.

There are some fun ideas coming down the road, and I believe the best ideas are yet to come. Heck, Vibrams were a boat shoe before they were discovered for running. Teva makes a split-toe sandal that may work well, and even Nike and Asics have their own split-toe shoes although they are no longer promoting them.

Who knows where the next great innovation will come from. Among the "little guys" out there we know about (and we're sure we're just scratching the surface), there's Sockwa, turning a beach sock into a running shoe; Heelus, a company in the UK exploring the idea of a shoe without a heel; Velocy, a company in the Northwest trying to build a shoe with a bigger or stiffer platform under the forefoot for greater stability and power.

And there's Dr. Craig Richards, a barefoot researcher who has taken it upon himself to develop a brand new type of sole (part of the shoe he calls the B.O.G. or barefoot on grass) that has scales that move independently like fish scales and let you feel the ground. There's also David Sypniewski in Florida, a barefoot runner, blogger, and enthusiast who's designing his own new shoe, the Skora.

I'm sure there are many, many more we don't even know about yet but who will make fantastic "strides" toward giving us healthier footwear that promotes a more natural stride.

I support all of these new designs. Some will work well, others won't, but by supporting them all we barefoot runners are helping change the industry and take footwear from antiquated fashion designs that hurt our feet to amazing, effective tools that help protect the feet and make us better.

With that said, I hope you explore the amazing range of new possibilities in footwear. Try them out, buy a pair or two, see which shoes you fall in love with. And promote, push, and support manufacturers and the little guys by voting with your dollars and your feet. Changing an industry isn't easy.

Together we can help change the world, the fitness of our youth, the peace of our minds, and the connection to our planet, one happy foot at a time.

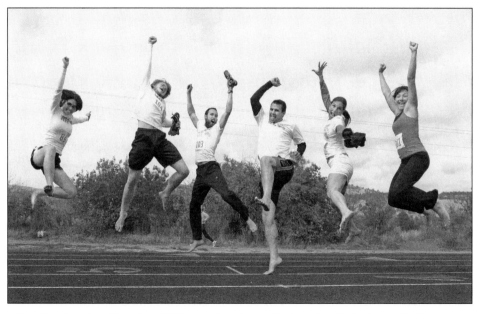

Boulder Barefoot Running Club members jump for joy after finishing a challenging race. Club founder, Jessica Lee, is on the left.

Part VI

The Final Step

We run, not because we think it is doing us good, but because we enjoy it and cannot help ourselves...The more restricted our society and work become, the more necessary it will be to find some outlet for this craving for freedom. No one can say, "You must not run faster than this, or jump higher than that." The human spirit is indomitable.

—Sir Roger Bannister

17

Barefoot for Life

Forget not that the earth delights to feel your bare feet and the winds long to play with your hair.

—Kahlil Gibran

I especially remember a morning when I was strolling past ivy leaves just as the sun began peeking out from behind some trees. One leaf held a tiny dew drop, and the first rays of the sun sliced through it and brought out all the colors of the rainbow. It was such a beautiful sight. I cried.

From that day on, I began looking at the world in a new way and started taking a camera with me on my runs. My photos have had gallery showings and have been purchased by art lovers around the world. They never would have happened if I hadn't slowed down long enough to see and appreciate the beauty all around me.

My skating accident taught me that a piano really can fall on our heads at any moment. And so the only path worth choosing is the one to happiness. And what made me happiest wasn't cycling, or skating, or hiking. It was running. And so with barefoot running I found a way to make my dreams come true.

My body is a living, breathing, constantly changing organism. And the trails I run on are alive and ever-changing as well—they bend, twist, ride up and plummet down in endless variations. How could anyone possibly make shoes that spontaneously react to such dynamic terrain?

I thought about the Native Americans who hundreds of years ago ran these same trails. They surely didn't wear orthotics or custom insoles in their moccasins. And yet they ran and ran and ran. And so we do too.

Our hope, as the minimalist trend and barefoot running take hold, not as a fad, but as a better way of doing things, it'll bring about a true renaissance in the sport. If you look around, chances are 99 out of 100 people loved running as a child, only to find it painful, boring, or tedious by the time they became adults. Now picture a world in which we all find running fun and exciting again.

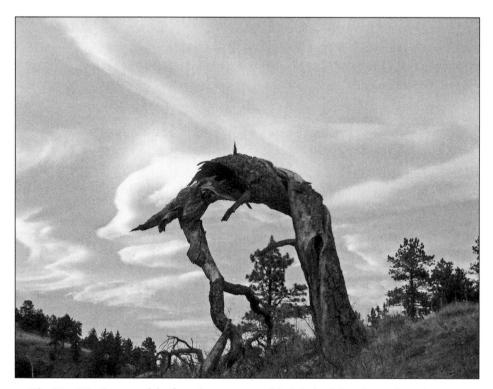

The "Zen Tree"—one of the first photos captured by Michael Sandler on his adventures out in nature to heal. His photography is now on display in galleries around the world. He credits nature and connecting with the earth for their beauty.

Running's a very green sport. There's little equipment, little impact, and when we're out on the trails, the last thing in the world we want to do is more harm to nature. When we connect to nature and to the earth, we view the world in a different way, and are constantly looking for new ways to reconnect and protect her.

Notes

[As of this printing, all links are accurate, but of course Internet links may change or disappear with time.]

Introduction

Memorial Day's Bolder Boulder is the second largest 10-kilometer race in the U.S., with over 40,000 participants annually, according to **http://racestats.blogspot .com/2005/05/bolder-boulder-10k.html**.

Orthopedic surgeon Dr. Joseph Froncioni's article, originally published in the German ultra magazine *Spiridon* in 2006 extolling the benefits of barefoot running started my profound journey. Read it and see for yourself: **www.runwithoutlimits.com/uploads/ATHLETIC_FOOTWEAR_AND_RUN NING_INJURIES.pdf.**

Chapter 1: Barefoot Running vs. Running with Shoes

Read about running's painful truths at **www.dailymail.co.uk/home/moslive/article -1170253/The-painful-truth-trainers-Are-expensive-running-shoes-waste-money .html**. This April 2009 article, "The Painful Truth about Trainers: Are Running Shoes a Waste of Money?" appears in the *MailOnline*.

The real truth about running shoes and cost: B. Marti, "Relationships Between Running Injuries and Running Shoes—Results of a Study of 5,000 Participants of a 16-km Run—The May 1984 Berne Grand Prix," in *The Shoe in Sport*, ed. B. Segesser and W. Pforringer, 256–265, Chicago: Year Book Medical Publishers, 1989.

More about running shoes and injuries in the definitive article by Dr. Joseph Froncioni at **www.runwithoutlimits.com/uploads/ATHLETIC_FOOTWEAR_AND_ RUNNING_INJURIES.pdf.**

The 1992 study of 2,300 Indian children that found that the chances of developing flat feet were over 3 times greater for the kids wearing shoes than for those going bare can be accessed here: U.B. Rao and B. Joseph, "The Influence of Footwear on the Prevalence of Flat Foot, a Survey of 2300 Children," *Journal of Bone and Joint Surgery* 74-B (July 1992): 525–527. See **www.jbjs.org.uk/cgi/reprint/74-B/4/525.pdf**.

For a thorough discussion of the evolution of barefoot running from a neuroanthropological viewpoint, see Greg Downey's article, "Lose Your Shoes: Is Barefoot Better" at **http://neuroanthropology.net/2009/07/26/lose-your-shoes-is-barefoot-better**.

For a more detailed discussion about how shoes may not only weaken feet but increase the chances of deforming them, see this article: B. Zipfel and L.R. Berger, "Shod Versus Unshod: The Emergence of Forefoot Pathology in Modern Humans?" *The Foot* 17 (2007): 205–213, doi:10.1016/j.foot.2007.06.002.

Preventing falls in the elderly—a discussion of injury prevention: N.D. Carter, P. Kannus, and K.M. Khan, "Exercise in the Prevention of Falls in Older People," *Sports Medicine* 31 (2001): 427–438. See **www.ncbi.nlm.nih.gov/pubmed/11394562.** Also, S. Robbins, E. Waked and J. McClaran, "Proprioception and Stability: Foot Position Awareness as a Function of Age and Footwear," *Oxford Journal of Age and Aging* (1995). See **http://ageing.oxfordjournals.org/cgi/content/abstract/24/1/67?ijkey=a d5b95ab57a716f394dda8b86279e3164c92ad44&keytype2=tf_ipsecsha.**

Chapter 6: Anatomy of the Barefoot Strike and Stride

Dr. Craig Richards, a researcher at the University of Newcastle in Australia, says it may take 6 months to learn to run barefoot as documented in the *British Journal of Sports Medicine*, via personal telephone conversation with the authors.

Dr. Marc Silberman, founder of the NJ Sports Medicine and Performance Center, comments on the difference between heel running and forefoot running in defining anatomically the hindfoot, midfoot, and forefoot. Although non-heel strike running has been called midfoot strike, this is incorrect and dangerous as most of the serious foot injuries occur in the midfoot (lisfranc sprain and navicular stress fracture); foot strike should occur in forefoot at metatarsal head/metatarsal phalangeal joint/pads.

The analogy comparing running in first and second gear is aided by thoughts from David Carrier, an evolutionary biologist at the University of Utah, in *Running Through the Ages* by Edward Sears.

Sakai, the Marathon Monk, is quoted from the book *The Marathon Monks of Mount Hiei* by John Stevens, p. 129.

Chapter 7: Turn Your Feet into Living Shoes

There are actually 28 bones in the foot, including 2 tiny bones called sesamoids located under the big toe joint, which are usually overlooked in the bone count, according to Dr. William A. Rossi, DPM, consultant to the footwear industry.

Chapter 8: Barefoot Runner Maintenance Tips and Tools

Plenty of helpful illustrations and photos: William A. Rossi, DPM, "Why Shoes Make 'Normal' Gait Impossible," *Podiatry Management* (March 1999), **http://nwfootankle .com/files/rossiWhyShoesMakeNormalGaitImpossible.pdf**

American Academy of Orthopaedic Surgeons, "If the Shoe Fits, Wear It." Order the free brochure at **http://orthoinfo.aaos.org/topic.cfm?topic=A00146**.

For more detailed definitions of arthritic conditions:
http://www.arthritis-guide.com/arthritis-glossary.htm.

Adaptation/injury prevention tidbits:
http://www.exrx.net/ExInfo/InjuryTidbits.html.

L. Klenerman and B. Wood, *The Human Foot: A Companion to Clinical Studies* (Springer, 2006), 45–48, 95–96.

The stick game is explained in Peter Nabakov's book, *Indian Running: Native American History and Tradition* (Ancient City Press, 1987).

This article in *Podiatry Today* talks about using tannic acid to toughen feet: Mark A. Caselli, CPM and Jean Chen-Vitulli, DPM, "Foot Blister Prevention: What You Can Recommend to Athletes," **http://www.podiatrytoday.com/article/291**, 15 (April 1, 2002).

Shin-Jung Park, Nori Kikufuji Ki-Ja Hyun and Hiromi Torkura, Hiromi, "Effects of Barefoot Habituation in Winter or Thermal and Hormonal Responses in Young Children—A Preliminary Study," *J Hum Ergology* 33 (2004): 61–67.

Chapter 9: On the Right Track with Nutrition

Ronald A. Hites and colleagues, "Global Assessment of Organic Contaminants in Farmed Salmon," *Science* 303 (2004) 226–229.

Deepak Chopra, *Magical Mind, Magical Body* (Nightingale Conant Corporation, 1994), audiobook.

Chapter 10: Weather or Not, Here I Come

For more on hyponatremia or overhydration, read this report from the Sports Research Intelligence Center, "Is Hydration Overrated?" by Matt Fitzgerald at:
http://sirc.ca/newsletters/july09/documents/21544220.pdf.

Another option for snow "shoes": I got this idea from Matt Carpenter, multi-time champion of the Pikes Peak Ascent and Marathon, and course record holder for the Leadville 100. He calls it the screw shoe (**http://www.skyrunner.com/screwshoe.htm**).

Chapter 12: Overcoming the Agony of the Feet

A study on plantar fasciitis by Lemont and colleagues found no inflammatory cells but degradation of the fascia, calling this plantar fasciosis or plantar fasciopathy. Others simply call it heel pain syndrome.

Li J and C. Muehleman, "Anatomic Relationship of Heel Spur to Surrounding Soft Tissue: Greater Variability than Previously Reported," *Clin Anat* 20 (2007): 950–955.

P. Jonsson and colleagues, "New Regimen for Eccentric Calf-Muscle Training in Patients with Chronic Insertional Achilles Tendinopathy: Results of a Pilot Study," *British Journal of Sports Medicine* 42 (2008): 746–749.

Chapter 14: Barefoot Children

Michael Nirenberg, "Footnotes," *NWI Parent* (July/Aug 2008): 20.

U.B. Rao and B. Joseph, "The Influence of Footwear on the Prevalence of Flat Foot, a Survey of 2300 Children," *Journal of Bone and Joint Surgery* 74-B (July 1992): 525–527. See www.jbjs.org.uk/cgi/reprint/74-B/4/525.pdf.

Michael Nirenberg, "What Are the Best Shoes for Children? The Answer May Surprise You." America's Podiatrist at: **http://www.americaspodiatrist.com/2009/12/what-are-the-best-shoes-for-chil dren-the-answer-may-surprise-you/**.

Shin-Jung Park, Nori Kikufuji Ki-Ja Hyun and Hiromi Torkura, Hiromi, "Effects of Barefoot Habituation in Winter or Thermal and Hormonal Responses in Young Children—A Preliminary Study," *J Hum Ergology* 33 (2004): 61–67, **http://sciencelinks .jp/j-east/article/200621/000020062106A0576685.php**.

Sebastian Wolf and colleagues, "Foot Motion in Children's Shoes: A Comparison of Barefoot Walking with Shod Walking in Conventional and Flexible Shoes," *Gait & Posture* 27 (2008): 51–59.

M. Walther and colleagues, "Children's Sport Shoes—A Systematic Review of Current Literature," *Foot Ankle Surg* 14 (2008): 180–189. Epub 2008 Jul 7.

Chapter 15: Barefoot Seniors Turn Back the Clock

Norman Doidge, *The Brain That Changes Itself: Stories of Personal Triumph from the Frontiers of Brain Science* (Penguin, 2007).

Gary Null and Amy McDonald. *Be a Healthy Women!* (Seven Stories Press, 2009), 527.

R.S. Rector and colleagues, "Participation in Road Cycling vs Running Is Associated with Lower Bone Mineral Density in Men," *Metabolism* 57 (2008): 226–232.

Joseph A. Buckwalter, "Decreased Mobility in the Elderly: The Exercise Antidote," *The Physician and Sportsmedicine* 25 (1997).

F. Li and colleagues, "Health Benefits from a Cobblestone-Mat Walking Activity: Findings from a Pilot Study," *Medicine & Science in Sports & Exercise* 35 (May 2003): S375.

Chapter 16: Minimalist Shoes and Other Essential Gear

A discussion of Dr. Marc Silberman's treadmill test in shoe selection by NJ Sports Medicine and Performance Center is at **http://njsportsmed.com**.

William A. Rossi, DPM, "Why Shoes Make 'Normal' Gait Impossible," Podiatry Management (March 1999) at **http://nwfootankle.com/files/rossiWhyShoesMake NormalGaitImpossible.pdf**.

Michael Nirenberg on sweating feet: **http://www.americaspodiatrist.com/2009/09/ can-the-color-of-your-shoes-affect-your-feet/**

About the Authors

Michael Sandler is a national fitness and running coach, as well as the cofounder of RunBare Company (www.RunBare.com). Michael has coached world-class athletes to wins in cycling, running, and triathlons for over 20 years at the local, national, and international levels.

Among Michael's personal athletic achievements are training for the 1992 and 1996 Olympics in both cycling and speed skating at the Olympic Training Center in Colorado Springs. While racing in Europe aiming for the Tour de France, an unexpected vehicle collision on a closed race-course dashed his chances for both international competitions.

Michael completed the California Ironman, and has a personal record for the 10K of 30:30 during the finishing leg of The Harvest Moon half-ironman. He went on to win a 2002 cycling state championship in Olympic sprints, beating the national team, and placed seventh in the master's national championships. In 2005, he garnered a sponsorship from Rollerblade for ultra-endurance inline speedskating. In 2009 he paced Barefoot Ted—a well-known, colorful figure in ultra-running—for the last leg of the Leadville 100, in which Ted shattered his own personal record by over an hour.

In 2004, Michael rode his bike in an entirely different direction. He completed a monumental bicycle trip across the U.S. by riding 5,000 miles in 40 days, solo and unsupported to raise awareness for children and adults with attention deficit disorder (ADD). He ended the ride in Washington, D.C., where he was invited to speak before the U.S. House and Senate on the Mental Health Parity Act, urging equal health coverage for psychological as well as physical health.

National and international media have interviewed him, including NPR, BBC, and America in the Morning. Michael has been featured on CNN, the CBS Early Morning Show in Chicago and New York for his athletic efforts to raise awareness of ADD.

He is also author of the best-selling book *College Confidence with ADD* and founder of The Creative Learning Institute, a national center for coaching students with ADD and learning disabilities.

In 2006, while training for a cross-country inline skating trip, Michael suffered a near-death accident, which left him with a shattered femur, hip, and arm. Michael surprised the medical community when he made a full recovery by running barefoot. Two months after the accident, he set the fastest record for the Bolder Boulder and Denver Half-Marathon by completing these popular races on crutches. He now runs barefoot 10 to 20 miles daily on rocky trails, hot asphalt, and even snow and ice, and sub-five minute miles barefoot all with his titanium femur and hip.

RunBare Company, based out of Boulder, holds clinics for barefoot running nationwide, and in Canada. Michael also conducts similar clinics for destination travel adventurists worldwide.

Jessica Lee holds a bachelor's degree in Learning and Organizational Change from Northwestern University's School of Education & Social Policy. Following graduation, she served two years with the U.S. Peace Corps as a Youth & Community Development volunteer in St. Vincent and the Grenadines. Her favorite project included launching a 4-H Club, which raised and sold chickens.

Back in the U.S., she spent a summer as a bicycle tour guide in Alaska before settling in Colorado where she became a jack of all trades, working as an REI Sales Specialist, managing a coffee shop, baking Italian artisan bread, and volunteering with Leave No Trace, a nonprofit that promotes environmental education and responsibility.

Eventually, Jessica settled into a focused career as a marketing professional in the renewable energy industry. In 2007, she ran the Bolder Boulder 10K and felt crippled with knee pain after the first 3K. After this unpleasant experience, she decided to give up the sport and focus her athletic efforts into cycling. This lasted until she met Michael and became inspired to run again, finding a pain-free joyous experience in barefoot running.

She went on to found the nation's largest barefoot running club in Boulder, followed by the co-founding of RunBare Company. Today she can be found running light and free again, and kicking Michael's butt in a sprint.

Together, Michael and Jessica enjoy starting each day with a barefoot sunrise hike and meditation before launching into the joyful work that lies ahead.

Resources

Books

Ali, Majid. *The Ghoraa and Limbic Exercise*. Life Span Books, 1993.

Brennan, J.H. *Tibetan Magic and Mysticism*. Llewellyn Publication, 2006.

Chopra, Deepak. *Magical Mind, Magical Body*. Nightingale Conant Corporation, 1994, audiobook.

Crowley, Chris, and Henry Lodge. *Younger Next Year: Live Strong, Fit, and Sexy—Until You're 80 and Beyond*. Workman, 2007.

Dispenza, Joe. *Evolve Your Brain: The Science of Changing Your Mind*. HCI, 2008.

Doidge, Norman. *The Brain That Changes Itself: Stories of Personal Triumph from the Frontiers of Brain Science*. Penguin, 2007.

Dreyer, Danny and Katherine Dreyer. *ChiRunning: A Revolutionary Approach to Effortless, Injury-Free Running*. Fireside, 2009.

Klenerman, L. and B. Wood. *The Human Foot: A Companion to Clinical Studies*. Springer, 2006.

Louv, Richard. *Last Child in the Woods: Saving Our Children from Nature-Deficit Disorder*. Algonquin Books, 2008.

McDougall, Christopher. *Born to Run: A Hidden Tribe, Superathletes, and the Greatest Race the World Has Never Seen*. Knopf, 2009.

Nabakov, Peter. *Indian Running: Native American History and Tradition*. Ancient City Press, 1987.

Nhat Hanh, Thich. *The Miracle of Mindfulness*. Beacon Press, 1999.

Noakes, Timothy. *The Lore of Running*. Human Kinetics, 2002.

Null, Gary and Amy McDonald. *Be a Healthy Women!* Seven Stories Press, 2009.

Poley, Rich and Tim Benko. *Self-Massage for Athletes*. Two Hands Press, 2007.

Romanov, Nicholas. *Dr. Nicholas Romanov's Pose Method of Running*. Pose Tech Press, 2004.

Rossi, William. *The Complete Footwear Dictionary*. Krieger, 2000; *The Sex Life of the Foot and Shoe*. Krieger, 1993.

Schaefer, Monika. *Reflexology Massage*. Sterling, 2008.

Sears, Edward. *Running Through the Ages*. McFarland, 2008.

Stevens, John. *The Marathon Monks of Mount Hiei*. Shambhala, 1988.

Miscellaneous Resources

Desert running phenom, Mike Stemple, is a serial entrepreneur. Gain confidence in whatever you do. Join his blog at **www.IamNotAfraid.com**.

Danny and Katherine Dreyer's revolutionary approach to effortless and injury-free running is spelled out in their best-selling book *ChiRunning* and in their clinics. Find out more at **www.chirunning.com**.

Christopher McDougall chronicled the greatest race the world has never seen in his astoundingly fascinating book, *Born to Run*. Two of those highly memorable, real-life characters can be reached at their Web sites: Take an adventure with Barefoot Ted McDonald at **www.barefootted.com**. He's contagious! And Caballo Blanco (Micah True) continues to donate and give back to the Raramuri (the "Tarahumara" or running people) in Mexico's Copper Canyons. Please consider donating too at **www .caballoblanco.com**.

Michael Sandrock helps so many people around the world with One World Running **http://oneworldrunning.blogspot.com**. Melody Varner is doing great work with helping Native American tribal members run their best at **www.nativerunners.org**.

YouTube Videos

Watch minimalist shoe reviews at **http://www.youtube.com/RunBareCompany**.

View Dr. Marc Silberman's running gait analysis videos at **http://www.njsportsmed .com./Video_Gait_Videos.html**.

Learn to treat your feet with self massage from Rich Poley, the author of *Self-Massage for Athletes* at **http://www.youtube.com/richpoley**.

Aids for Relaxation and Getting Grounded

Earth Songs: Mountains, Water and the Healing Power of Nature, a documentary produced by stress expert Brian Luke Seaward, narrated by actor Michael York with music composed by Academy Award–winning composer, Brian Keane, is a breathtaking symphony of life that invites us all to renew our relationship with nature. *Earth Songs* was made as a relaxation DVD. Visit **http://brianlukeseaward.net**. Preview on You-Tube at **www.youtube.com/watch?v=swE5aYurZcg**.

Feel better, sleep better with grounding pads. Learn more from our expert Dale Teplitz at **www.barefoothealth.com.**

Tools for Conditioning

Explore RunBare products such as balls and Barefoot Beads at **www.RunBare.com.**

Start your feet and ankles on the path to recovery with Correct Toes at **www .nwfootankle.com.** Realigning your toes as nature intended realigns your body for better balance and stride.

If you're in Boulder, Colorado, stop in at In-Step, a minimalist friendly footwear shop, or check it out online at **www.instepbldr.com.**

Visit **www.InvisibleShoe.com** for a modern day take of huaraches, the traditional Mexican running sandals of the Tarahumara.

Acknowledgments

Whenever you see a book, you're seeing the tip of the iceberg. Like a duck serenely moving on water, there's major paddling going on beneath the surface. This is where we pull the paddlers to the surface and thank them.

This book could not have existed without the assistance, guidance, and love of so many others. We say love because there's been such incredible warmth and compassion in the help we've received. This book truly is a labor of love by all who've been involved.

Mike Stemple is a "Serial Entrepreneur" and desert running phenom whose real-world experience and unabashed guidance gave us the wherewithal, direction, and confidence to pursue this project. R.L. Smith and Tricia Vieth told Michael, "Maybe you just don't belong in shoes," and that helped spark the epiphany about barefoot running. With your desire to help runners, we know your minimalist footwear shop called In-Step in Boulder will be a great success.

To Danny Dreyer, author of *ChiRunning*, your work has helped countless thousands of runners and your amazing foreword and beautiful words are the perfect start to this book. Barefoot Ted McDonald poured out his contagious youthful spirit. And Caballo Blanco (Micah True), you've helped keep us on the straight and narrow. We hope more people visit your site (**www.caballoblanco.com**) and your race to donate and give back to the Raramuri (the "Tarahumara" or running people).

Steven Sashen and Lena Phoenix dished out invaluable entrepreneurial and SEO advice. Zach Bergen lent us his brilliant mind and loving spirit. Paul Weppler aka "The Rock Hopper," we thank you for your consummate out-of-the-box thinking, assistance, and killer massage skills. Thanks to David Fox for challenging us to take a good long look at the future.

Our medical advisers brought a wealth of insight and foresight. Dr. Marc and Amy Silberman shared their insightful knowledge and fantastic YouTube videos. Dr. Lisa Harner provided pediatric and professional dancing expertise. Neuroplastician Dr. Michael Merzenech helped us wrap our minds around mapping the mind. Keeping us grounded and explaining the physics was Dale Teplitz, M.A. Dr. Craig Richards and Dr. Daniel Lieberman shared their research findings on barefoot running. And Dr. David Carrier explained the evolutionary research into how we came to be a running species.

Our book production team brought their expertise to the words and pictures. Sandra Wendel, the world's most expedient, effective, and organized editor, we thank you for holding our hands and walking us through this process. To Gregory Fields—for pulling off a layout miracle and for taking our ideas and translating them into a beautiful reality. Hy Bender got us started and kept the "bloated whale" (aka first draft) from sinking.

We thank Kennan Harvey for our cover photo and Web site shots and for not getting Michael killed when trying to climb down off an arch. Josephine Pham's photos appear in this book. Her pictures are worth more than a thousand words. Thanks go to Ray Keller for his amazing video skills under the most trying of conditions such as filming in a snowstorm. Jack Burden's strong guidance and occasional kick in the butt spurred us on our way.

To the great folks at the Boulder Recreation Center who let us use their facilities. Special thanks to Dr. Michael Wertz for putting Michael back together. Becky Hearty, an inspirational physical therapist when it was needed most and to everyone at Boulder Community Hospital.

Michael Sandrock, has helped so many people around the world with his non-profit One World Running. To Melody Varner for sharing her wisdom on Native American running and for her great work in helping tribal runners reach their full potential. Pam Guyton and Jan Dunn, for their Franklin Method and Pilates wisdom that has helped athletes learn to move their bodies with ease and comfort. To Dr. William A. Weber, author of *Colorado Flora* (Eastern and Western Slope volumes) for your playful glee on the cobblestone mat at the ever young age of 91. By staying active and writing, you're showing us all how to stay young of body and of mind.

Crazy Bob, you're still the man! To Hendrick Maako for his friendship and sharing his wealth of knowledge on growing up running barefoot. Dennis Shaver and Joey Barbosa, who supported us from the very beginning. Scott McLean for his overflowing exuberance and everyone in the barefoot running club in Boulder, Colorado. Shota Shikata for your friendship and valiant efforts, you're an agent for change, and you'll go far!

To Jessica's father, William Lee, for believing in our mission. Without his support, this entire project would have been stuck on the ground.

To our families and especially, Michael's sister, Elisa Sandler, thank you for your enthusiasm and gung-ho attitude. Aliya Sternstein for early editorial guidance. Diane Byrne "meow-meow," for brutal editorial prowess and everyone else who read the manuscript in advance and offered advice.

To the anonymous father and toddler who stepped out on Michael's path, the accident that followed helped bring him here today. Everything truly happens for a reason.

To God and the Universe, thank you for driving the ship. None of this would have been possible without God's grace, love, compassion, and guidance.

Index